COMMON SKIN DISORDERS

A Physician's Illustrated Manual
With Patient Instruction Sheets

2nd Edition

Ernst Epstein, M.D.

MEDICAL ECONOMICS BOOKS
Oradell, New Jersey 07649

Library of Congress Cataloging in Publication Data

Epstein, Ernst.
   Common skin disorders

   Includes index.
   1. Skin—Diseases—Handbooks, manuals, etc.
I. Title. [DNLM: 1. Skin diseases. WR 140 E6304]
RL74.E67 1983   616.5   82-14254
ISBN 0-87489-308-9 (pbk.)

Design by Penny Seldin

ISBN 0-87489-308-9

Medical Economics Company Inc.
Oradell, New Jersey 07649

First Edition   1979
Second Edition   1983

Printed in the United States of America

To my wife, Jan, and our son, Steve—
for their love, understanding, and patience

Contents

Foreword

Dermatology is a deceptive specialty—it appears a simple matter of looking at spots and prescribing ointments. Nothing could be farther from the truth: I've practiced dermatology for two decades and remain amazed at the complexities of diagnosis and treatment.

Ernst Epstein has spent several years refining his clinical practices, including the information and instruction sheets for patients. Here he summarizes his knowledge succinctly in a practical"how-to" text for both physicians and patients.

Some physicians might, at first, consider this approach too impersonal. If, however, you and your staff use the patient instruction sheets systematically, you'll find they actually give you a more personal approach to patient care. By freeing you from the boring repetition of routine information, these instruction sheets will give you more time to discuss your patients' individual needs.

Dermatology is continually changing. You can easily and inexpensively update the instruction sheets to incorporate advances in diagnosis and treatment. The role of this book in patient care should be many times its size.

Howard Maibach, M.D.
Professor of Dermatology
University of California
Medical Center
San Francisco

Preface to the second edition

Dermatology is primarily a visual science, so the incorporation of color photographs in this second edition will enhance its clinical value. The photographs were chosen to emphasize diagnostic and therapeutic points in common, treatable conditions that may go unrecognized by the general physician. Four new sections, dealing with dermatofibromas, keloids, molluscum contagiosum, and nevi, have been added. The surgery chapter has been expanded to describe skin closure with gut sutures, which eliminate the need for patients to return for suture removal. Recent advances in therapy required updating of several sections and extensive rewriting of the acne unit. Throughout, I have attempted to emphasize the simplest and best current therapy for each disorder.

Ernst Epstein, M.D.

Preface to the first edition

Many skin diseases are chronic; some are incurable. Patients' comfort and appearance depend on following treatment instructions accurately and intelligently. Upon beginning private practice, therefore, I wrote a treatment outline for each patient. Not only did these written summaries reassure my patients, they also improved treatment results. As other physicians have done, I had some of the more common instructions printed in volume. These printed sheets proved so useful that their number increased to more than 30 and they became an essential part of my practice. Colleagues visiting my office liked the systematic use of instruction sheets; several suggested their wider dissemination. Thus was born the idea of this book.

A collection of instruction sheets by itself, however, would have left out someone very important—you. Hence the portions of this book directed to the nonspecialist in dermatology who needs practical pointers on therapy—the small but essential details the textbooks omit.

Dermatology texts also tend to offer a potpourri of possible therapies for each disease. Which to choose? The ones I like best: the treatments I've found to be most successful, easiest for patients, and, when possible, least expensive. Where there's controversy, I've explained why I believe one treatment is better than another. And, because this book is intended primarily for the nondermatologist, I've included only the more common skin disorders.

Medicine can be a most rewarding profession. Often it's frustrating. The conscientious clinician is caught between the ideal of perfect medicine and the realities of limited time, knowledge, patients' understanding, and compliance. By sharing with you and your patients some of the therapeutic techniques I've found helpful, I hope to help overcome some of these limitations.

Ernst Epstein, M.D.

Acknowledgments

Dr. Howard Maibach provided the stimulus to write this book. He generously read the preliminary manuscript and contributed valuable guidance and advice as well as the foreword. Janice Crossman and Kathy Henne of my office staff were innovative in utilizing the instruction forms and made many helpful suggestions. For this revised edition, their assistance with taking photographs was invaluable. The editorial staff of Medical Economics Books guided me through the steps of writing and revising a book. Their upbeat correspondence was constantly encouraging. For the many typings and revisions I am grateful to my secretary, Natalie Bowhay.

I am indebted to the publishers of *Cutis* for permission to reprint Tables 12-1 and 12-2 in the unit on hand dermatitis.

Publisher's notes

Ernst Epstein, M.D., earned his master's degree in biochemistry as well as his doctorate in medicine at Marquette University. After his residency at the University of Pennsylvania Hospital, he became affiliated with the San Mateo, California, Medical Clinic. Since 1971 he has engaged in the private practice of dermatology in San Mateo.

Dr. Epstein is clinical associate professor of dermatology at the University of California, San Francisco, Medical Center. His professional publications have appeared in the *Journal of the American Medical Association*, *Archives of Dermatology*, the *British Journal of Dermatology*, and *Cutis*.

Introduction:
How to use this book

This book is for the physician and his/her assistants who treat skin diseases. It is not a textbook—absent are the complete disease descriptions that characterize dermatologic texts. Instead you are provided specific, detailed treatment directions for common skin disorders. I present what appears to be the best single therapy, rather than a bewildering array of possible remedies. The choice of "best" approach reflects my prejudices favoring simplicity, safety, and proven efficacy; some arbitrariness is unavoidable. Where controversies exist, I explain the reason for my position. When there is no effective therapy—as in herpes simplex—this unpleasant fact is stated.

Units covering skin diseases commonly encountered in North America make up the core of this book. For each disease there's a patient information sheet—sometimes more than one—and a unit for the physician that details therapy. The patient instruction sheet is meant to be copied and given to the patient as an integral part of medical management. These patient information sheets make for more effective therapy, please patients, and save the physician's time.

This introduction describes how the book, particularly the patient information sheets, can be employed for increased effectiveness in treating skin disorders. The following three chapters take up subjects of particular interest in treating skin diseases: topical corticosteroids, diagnosing dermatitis, and dermatologic surgical techniques.

Specialist and generalist both will find this book useful. The introductory chapters and the physician portion of each disease unit were written with the nonspecialist in mind. The patient instruction sheets should appeal to all clinicians who treat skin diseases. Many physicians would make use of them if they were available. Here they are.

The patient instruction sheet

Communicating with patients

All clinicians know that successful patient management requires the patient's cooperation. Patients will cooperate fully only if they understand what they have to do, and why. Medical problems may be complex, and patients often fail to understand them. Finally, if the physician relies exclusively on the spoken word to inform and instruct patients, they're all too likely to forget what he said.

How quickly talk is forgotten! We all took copious notes during our professional training. Astute businessmen invariably confirm a verbal discussion or agreement with a written memo. Yet most physicians rely on purely verbal communication to present difficult concepts and unfamiliar instructions. Patients' ability to remember is further impaired by the anxiety most experience in a doctor's office. Little wonder that patients complain they didn't understand what they were told, and remember less of that!

Our knowledge works against us here. Without thinking, we use terms that we don't consider technical—*lesion, benign, dermatitis*—with no inkling that they're sailing over the patient's head. We take for granted that patients understand many disorders are idiopathic and chronic. Not so. Patients desire simple explanations as to causes, and they expect cures for their illnesses. Nor do we consider patients' concerns and fears: Who routinely reassures a new patient with psoriasis that it is not contagious and that the lesions are not cancerous? These concepts are of such second nature to us that they don't enter our minds. Yet such worries may lie heavily on a patient's mind.

The inadequacy of talk as the sole means of communicating with patients is obvious. How about writing out the necessary information? Many physicians do write a summary of instructions for patients. Time pressure and the quality of most doctors' handwriting limit the usefulness of this method. It's impossible for even the most conscientious physician to cover all matters relating to every patient complaint—but it isn't impossible to set all this information down clearly once, have it reproduced, and hand it to patients.

Patients love information sheets

At least once daily a patient tells me, "These information sheets are great." Then they continue, "Why don't other doctors use them?" Many needless fears are alleviated when an information sheet is reread and digested away from the anxiety-producing doctor's office. Teen-agers feel less guilty about their acne after learning it is not the result of poor skin hygiene. Parents stop worrying that their children's eczema results from inadequate care. Patients with psoriasis understand that it is not contagious and feel free to approach their mates sexually.

What might seem a minor misunderstanding to us may lead to major patient concerns. One elderly, retired skin-cancer patient is deeply grateful, not for my treatment of his skin cancers, but because he again feels free to play golf. His previous—and competent—dermatologist told him that skin cancers resulted from sun damage and he should avoid the sun. Being conscientious, the patient took this literally and gave up his favorite recreation since he recognized that it was impossible to play golf without sun exposure. Upon reading the information sheets on skin cancer and sun protection he learned that it's the *cumulative* effect of sunlight over many years that does the damage, and that moderate amounts of sun exposure add little harm. After reading these instructions, he resumed his golf game and made a point of expressing his pleasure. Without the information sheets, this problem would never have come to my attention.

Why you will like these patient instruction sheets

In addition to pleasing patients, these instruction sheets will save you time, eliminate most repetitive questions, and decrease telephone calls. They simplify the management of complex as well as routine dermatologic problems.

For example: 17-year-old John comes to have his wart removed; he has his parents' permission but is alone. You explain that the wart is a harmless nuisance easily removed by minor surgery, and remove it. Then John is given the superficial skin surgery instructions and requested to read them several times as they tell him how to care for the scab. He's told that warts are caused by a virus and is given the wart information sheet to read at home. You ask John to show both sheets to his parents. Result: John cares for his wound properly and there's no follow-up telephone call from a parent asking whether the wound can be gotten wet, whether it must be bandaged, whether warts can turn cancerous, and so on.

Another example: 14-year-old Mary, accompanied by her mother, consults you for her acne. When they're taken into the treatment room, they're each given the acne information sheet and asked to read it while waiting for the doctor. After allowing enough time for them to assimilate it, you enter, take the history, and examine Mary. The instruction sheet has answered most questions, and you can concentrate on specific problems (why do you pick?) and therapy. Since the patient information sheet answers routine questions, you're saved the boredom of repeatedly answering the same questions.

A week later you see Mary's mother (impressed by your patient information sheets) for a troublesome hand dermatitis that's failed to respond to numerous home remedies. You diagnose an irritant (housewife's) hand dermatitis and instruct her in hand protection by going over major points of the hand protection sheet. You ask her to read the sheet once daily at home for three days. Here an instruction sheet is not just a convenient timesaver; it's an essential part of treatment. No patient could remember half this advice if you gave it verbally, even if you had the time.

Next you hand Mary's mother a hand dermatitis treatment sheet and ask her to read it while you're writing a prescription for a topical corticosteroid. You show her how to apply topicals properly, go over the major points (no hand lotions or home remedies), and ask her to reread the instructions at home. Success in treating hand dermatitis often hinges on careful attention to details—far too many to be entrusted to the fragile human memory.

How to use patient instruction sheets

The preceding examples illustrate how patient information sheets can be integrated into medical practice. It is not a case of making a diagnosis, handing the patient a prescription and information sheet, and sending him on his way. The patient information sheets supplement and expand verbal explanations. Treatment for many dermatologic conditions is highly individualized; therefore the treatment instructions in many patient sheets are general. Specific instructions for each patient should be written on the information sheet. Some sheets have blank spaces in which you can write the name of the medication you prescribe or recommend. Some parts of information sheets may be irrelevant and should be crossed off.

Patient sheets provide a mixture of information and treatment instructions. Some, like the psoriasis sheet, provide mainly background information. Others, such as the various postoperative sheets, consist entirely of specific treatment instructions. Being aware of these two elements will help you make optimal use of patient sheets.

Sheets containing primarily information are useful—

1. To provide general information before the patient is seen. If the patient has a readily recognized complaint, such as warts or acne, reading the patient sheet will provide information that otherwise would require additional physician time.
2. To inform the patient after he is examined. When examination discloses a condition such as psoriasis, alopecia areata, scabies, or atopic eczema, the patient is told the diagnosis and asked to read the information sheet after getting dressed. I add that I will return to provide treatment instructions and answer any questions. This technique is especially useful if the patient has a disorder that's unfamiliar (e.g., alopecia areata) or widely misunderstood (e.g., scabies). I use this technique when patients return for treatment of a biopsy-proven basal-cell carcinoma. They're given the basal-cell cancer sheet to read before I see them. My preoperative explanation can then focus on the treatment technique, sutures, scarring, and other problems.
3. As a reasonable way of dealing with "by the way" questions. For example, you've just removed a wart from the forefinger of a 28-year-old, fair-skinned woman. As you prepare to dismiss her, she asks if sunlight is bad for her skin and whether she should avoid it. Her reason for asking? Her father had several skin cancers and told her sunlight caused them. Here's an excellent opportunity to practice preventive medicine by spending 10 or 15 minutes discussing solar damage and sun-protective measures. Are you willing to wreck your schedule that way—or do you brush her question off by stating that sunlight *is* bad for the skin and should be avoided? An effective approach is to agree that sunlight damages the skin and then add—while handing her the sheet titled "Sunlight and Your Skin"—"This sheet explains it and gives you specific advice on how to prevent sun damage to your skin. Please read it carefully at home."

This technique is useful when patients raise questions not related to their own care. Dad wants to know if his teen-age Billy has pimples because he isn't washing his face enough. It turns out that the few pimples aren't bothering Billy, but the face-washing issue has triggered a family war. You reassure Dad that dirt does not cause pimples, give him the acne sheet to read at home, and add, "If Billy's acne does become troublesome, bring him in."

Primarily "operational" sheets are useful—

1. For routine postoperative care.
2. For performing standard but detailed treatments. Examples are the sheets on hand dermatitis, hand protection, plantar warts, and chemical destruction of warts. Since the treatment varies little from case to case, it can be presented in a standard printed form.

Mechanics: Reproduction and storage

The patient instruction sheets are meant to be copied and given to the patient. For occasional use, photocopies are fine; when larger numbers are needed, offset printing by one of the many rapid printing shops is cheap and fast. Since offset printing uses photocopying techniques, either way of producing copies enables you to alter them by changing the master copy.

Personalize the instruction sheets by adding your name and telephone number. Changes are easy. You can provide additional information by adding a paragraph. Parts of the master can be blocked off with opaque paper; they will appear blank on the copies. An outdated section can be cut out, a new version typed, and the master put together with double-sided paper-mending tape; the surgery won't show in the copies. There will be a difference in type with this method of change; if that annoys you, have a new master typed.

Keep a supply of instruction sheets in each examining room so you can quickly hand your patient the appropriate one. A file cabinet is ideal for storage; if there's no space for one, an expandable compartmented manila file folder works well. Ready availability is important: If the sheets are stored outside the examining room, it will often be too much trouble to get them.

Writing your own

Every physician should have an information sheet introducing himself and his practice to new patients. While some offices provide printed booklets, a typed sheet is simple and adequate. Physicians' practices vary so widely that it must be written by you. Check with colleagues in your field and ask to borrow parts of their new patient sheets that you like, or use the example* in this chapter to get ideas.

Your new-patient information sheet should briefly describe the nature of your practice and provide specifics as to office hours, appointments, emergency coverage, fees and payment, insurance forms, and anything else your

---

*I am indebted to David Harris, M.D., for large portions of this information sheet for new patients.

new patients should know. If yours is a group practice, describe your coverage procedure. Keep it short!

Using patient information sheets is habit-forming. They work so well you'll soon want more. Write your own, using simple words and short sentences. Have your effort read carefully by a nonmedical person who isn't afraid to criticize your writing. It should come back full of suggested changes and half as long. If it doesn't, either you have a remarkable knack for clear writing or you've chosen the wrong person to criticize your efforts.

Have a master copy of the final version typed, and test it by giving patients photocopies. If the sheets prove worthy and larger numbers are needed, have the master reproduced by offset printing.

To sum up the practical points:

1. Keep it short.
2. Use simple language and short sentences.
3. Keep descriptions of therapy sufficiently general so that minor changes won't make your sheet obsolete. When some new, superior fungicides were marketed recently, I had to discard a batch of tinea cruris instructions since they named an older, less effective fungicide in the treatment section.
4. Find a critical editor to proofread your efforts.
5. Try to leave space at the bottom of the sheet to write specific instructions.
6. Revise your sheet to keep up with new developments and when you see a chance to present material more clearly.

Leslie P. Dexter, M.D., Inc.
Dermatology
487 Richardsville Road
San Mateo, Calif. 94401
Telephone (415) 555-1234

NEW-PATIENT INFORMATION

Please keep for future reference

1. MY SPECIALTY

My practice is limited to dermatology. I am a board-certified specialist trained to diagnose and treat skin diseases. These conditions range from acne to warts. They include diseases of hair and nails.

2. REGISTRATION

Our receptionist will ask you to fill out a registration form for recording your history, findings, and treatment. Please print your full name, including your middle name, and exact date of birth. If you were referred by another doctor, please indicate this so we can send him a report.

3. INITIAL VISIT

Your first visit begins with a history of your skin problem. Next is a careful examination of your skin. The nature of your problem and suggested treatment will be discussed with you.

4. OFFICE HOURS

Patients are seen *by appointment only,* during office hours: 8:00 to 12:00 Mondays, Tuesdays, Thursdays, and Fridays, 2:15 to 5:00 Mondays, Tuesdays, Wednesdays, and Fridays. For *emergencies* we are available at all times through our answering service.

5. TELEPHONE CALLS

An assistant is available to answer your calls from 7:45 to 12:30 and 1:30 to 5:00. To change or cancel an appointment *please call during office hours* **at least 24 hours prior to your appointment.** Before or after office hours, our answering service will take your call.

6. PRESCRIPTIONS

Please take your prescription to the pharmacy of your choice. For accuracy, you are given written prescriptions; we do *not* telephone in prescriptions. The pharmacist will label each prescription with the name of the medication and directions for using it. Medications that are refillable will be marked with the number of refills allowed. You can obtain a refill by returning the container to the *same pharmacy* or using the prescription number on the container. This office has one unyielding policy: Prescriptions will be refilled only if you have been seen in the office within the last 12 months.

7. FEES AND BILLING

At the end of your visit, you will be given a small yellow slip to be taken to the receptionist. This slip indicates the time of your next appointment, the type of medical service, and the fee. You may pay at the time of each visit or be billed, whichever you prefer. (Nonresidents are expected to pay at each visit.) Initial visit fees depend on the complexity of the problem and the amount of time required. Return visits are usually $25.

Office surgery is billed separately. If your visit is for office surgery, only a charge for surgery is made. The fee includes a brief, no-charge checkup visit.

8. PAYMENT FOR SERVICES

Medical services are charged directly to you, not your insurance company. Patients are personally responsible for paying their medical bills. Payment is due on receipt of statement.

You are responsible for paying your bill in full even if insurance benefits are pending. If your insurance check gets sent to us, any overpayment will be returned to you. We cannot accept the responsibility for collecting your insurance claim or negotiating a settlement on a disputed claim.

Should you have questions about the fee, or any problems with payment, please discuss this with me or one of my assistants.

9. INSURANCE

Our policy is for patients to process all insurance forms themselves. You will receive an itemized bill in duplicate and a blue instruction sheet telling you how to prepare insurance claims. The bill shows the diagnosis in a standard code, the treatment you received, the date of service, and the charge. This is all the *medical* information the insurance companies require. Submit your claim, following the directions on the blue sheet, and enclose one copy of your bill—the other copy is for your records. The insurer will then reimburse *you* for medical costs covered by your policy. The doctor's signature is NOT needed on your insurance forms.

This procedure has significantly shortened the time our patients wait for reimbursement from insurance carriers.

Should you have problems or questions in filing your insurance claims, we will be happy to assist you.

10. HOW YOU CAN HELP US

When you must cancel or change an appointment, please call us 24 hours *in advance.* Please notify us of a change in your address or telephone number.

Rational use of topical corticosteroids | 1

Topical corticosteroids are the most commonly prescribed agents in dermatologic treatment. They are remarkably effective for numerous—but by no means all—disorders.[1-3] Many physicians use them on a trial-and-error basis. This is unfortunate, as the effectiveness of topical corticosteroid therapy can usually be predicted if you consider (1) the disorder that is being treated, (2) the site, (3) the potency of the preparation, and (4) the nonspecific effects of the vehicle.

Role of the disorder in determining corticosteroid therapy

Topical corticosteroids are the sovereign remedy for a wide variety of eczematous dermatoses, including atopic dermatitis, asteatotic eczema, nummular eczema, and the many eczematous dermatoses that don't fit conventional classifications. Pruritus vulvae and idiopathic pruritus ani usually respond. Contact dermatitis is responsive to topical corticosteroids in the subacute and chronic stages, when swelling has diminished. In the acute edematous and vesicular stages, topical corticosteroids are ineffective. Stasis dermatitis improves with topical corticosteroids; additional treatment of the venous stasis is usually necessary for satisfactory control.

The response of psoriasis to topical corticosteroids varies with the individual and the skin site. Intertriginous (skin-fold) psoriasis responds well to topical corticosteroids, while the response of glabrous (smooth) skin is variable and scalp psoriasis responds to topical corticosteroids only if the scale is first removed. The corticosteroid must be carefully matched with the site.

While topical corticosteroids are of benefit in certain infrequent disorders such as discoid lupus erythematosus, most other disorders respond poorly or not at all.

Role of the skin site

Topical corticosteroids are most effective in intertriginous areas, have an intermediate effect on glabrous skin, and are least effective on the palms and soles. In general, efficacy parallels their percutaneous penetration. The scalp may be an exception; while corticosteroids are readily absorbed through scalp skin, many scalp dermatoses respond poorly to topical corticosteroids. Side effects accompany benefits; skin atrophy and striae from topical corticosteroids occur most rapidly in skin-fold areas.

The differing responses of skin sites are of practical importance. Low-potency corticosteroids, such as 1 or 2 per cent hydrocortisone, are preferred for skin-fold areas since they usually produce an adequate response with little risk of skin atrophy. Corticosteroids of intermediate potency will often be necessary on glabrous skin; the face is an exception, as it usually responds well to low-potency corticosteroids. Palms and soles require the most potent corticosteroids, often with occlusion to increase their effectiveness.

The site influences the choice of vehicle. On the hairy scalp, creams and ointments tend to make the hair a greasy mess. Solutions, gels, and aerosol sprays are best for treating hairy areas. While it's possible to apply almost any type of vehicle to other skin areas, ointments are often poorly tolerated in skin-fold areas. Dermatitis of skin folds is better treated with a cream or lotion. On glabrous skin, the choice of vehicle will be determined by the acuteness of the dermatitis and by the effect desired—drying or lubricating.

Potency of topical corticosteroid preparations

There are great differences in the potencies of commercial topical corticosteroid formulations, which range from the weak 0.5 per cent hydrocortisone cream* to highly potent fluorinated compounds. The potency of corticosteroids depends on three variables: (1) the molecular structure, (2) the concentration, and (3) the vehicle.

1. Corticosteroids differ in their anti-inflammatory effects. For example, topically triamcinolone acetonide is many times as potent as hydrocortisone. Not all the newer corticosteroids are superior to hydrocortisone in topical usage. The relative effectiveness of these drugs can be determined only by careful paired comparison trials in a variety of steroid-responsive dermatoses—a tedious task. We don't yet have such data for many of the newer corticosteroid preparations.

2. The role of concentration in determining potency is recognized by many manufacturers, who produce preparations of varying concentrations. Hydrocortisone concentrations of less than 1 per cent are an obsolete heritage from times when the drug was costly. Triamcinolone acetonide preparations are marketed in concentrations of 0.025, 0.1, and 0.5 per cent. The 0.025 per cent triamcinolone acetonide concentration is adequate for most uses; stubborn dermatoses may yield to the 0.5 per cent concentration.

---

*In the United States, 0.5 per cent hydrocortisone topical preparations are available without a prescription. They have a weak effect and may control minimal to mild atopic or seborrheic dermatitis. However, many persons use it for various acute processes where it is of no value or—in the case of pyodermas—actually contraindicated.

3. The vehicle plays an important role in determining potency. Corticosteroid creams were first prepared by dispersing the drug in a water-washable cream base, while a petrolatum base was used for ointments. The greasy ointment is usually more potent than the cream. Topical corticosteroids are most potent when dissolved in the vehicle with propylene glycol or a similar solvent. Specialized corticosteroid vehicles should not be mixed with other topical agents, creams, or ointments, as the unique effect of the vehicle may be destroyed.

The technique of solubilizing corticosteroids in their vehicles has led manufacturers to upgrade their older preparations by revising the vehicles. Result: a bewildering set of new trade preparations. Fluocinolone is sold by Syntex as Synalar (old base) and as Synemol when incorporated in the new base. Lederle has revised its triamcinolone formulation so there is Aristocort (old) and Aristocort A (new formulation)—to name only two manufacturers. Because of higher solvent concentrations, some newer cream and gel vehicles are more irritating than older ointment bases, especially when occluded.

Table 1-1 provides a rough classification of the potencies of some of the topical corticosteroids most commonly used in the United States. To avoid a myriad of names, I omitted many topical corticosteroids that, although effective, have no real advantage over older preparations.

The relative potencies of corticosteroids may differ depending upon the disease treated. Thus, many of the newer fluorinated formulations provide similar excellent results in atopic dermatitis but show significant variation in their effects on psoriasis. Acquaint yourself thoroughly with a few topical

TABLE 1-1

Rough guide to the relative potencies of some commonly used corticosteroids

POTENCY	GENERIC NAME	TRADE NAME(S)	STRENGTH
Highest	Triamcinolone acetonide	Aristocort, Kenalog	0.5%
	Fluocinonide	Lidex, Topsyn	0.05%
	Halcinonide	Halog	0.1%
High	Betamethasone valerate	Valisone	0.1%
	Triamcinolone acetonide	Aristocort, Kenalog	0.1%
Intermediate	Triamcinolone acetonide	Aristocort, Kenalog	0.025%
	Flurandrenolide	Cordran	0.025%
	Fluocinolone	Synalar	0.01*%
	Desonide	Tridesilon	0.05%
	Hydrocortisone		3-5%
Low	Hydrocortisone		1%

*Also available in 0.025 per cent strength. The 0.01 per cent strength is intermediate in potency.

Topical corticosteroids

corticosteroid formulations. Prescribe only one or two preparations in each category rather than order the latest miracle detailed by salesmen or glowingly advertised.

Nonspecific effects of the vehicle

The type of vehicle—ointment, cream, lotion, gel, solution, or aerosol—has a significant nonspecific effect on dermatitis. Prior to corticosteroids, treatment of dermatitis depended chiefly on such nonspecific effects. Although the nonspecific effects of a vehicle are less important now, they play a significant—and often underappreciated—role in treating dermatitis.

The aim of the vehicle is to help normalize dermatitic skin. Solutions and gels generally have a drying effect; greasy ointments have a pronounced lubricating effect. Creams and lotions have a slight lubricating effect. Physicians often err in relying on just one type of preparation—usually a cream— to treat all corticosteroid-responsive dermatoses. Cream preparations are ideal for most acute and subacute rashes but not for dry, fissuring dermatoses, which do best with ointments. Ointments are messier than creams, although if applied thinly they're usually acceptable. In more acute processes an ointment's occlusive effect may irritate; creams or lotions are usually better choices. Even an experienced dermatologist may be in doubt as to what vehicle will produce the best response. A simple solution is to have the patient apply a corticosteroid cream to one site and the same drug in ointment form to a matched contralateral site. Any significant difference in effectiveness will be evident in a few days.

Other considerations in prescribing

Cost

There are significant cost differences between corticosteroids of approximately equal potency. Many of the newer fluorinated preparations are much more expensive than the correspondingly potent triamcinolone acetonides. Some brands of 1 per cent hydrocortisone are double the cost of others. The difference can be significant to patients who may need several refills. When prescribing hydrocortisone topicals, you can save your patients money by writing generically. Spend a few minutes comparing prices in your pharmacist's book of wholesale costs. As a basic intermediate-strength corticosteroid, 0.025 per cent triamcinolone acetonide is usually the best buy.

How much to prescribe?

How much corticosteroid to prescribe depends on the patient's needs, the price, and the packaging. If the patient applies his corticosteroid sparingly, his needs can be estimated accurately. The amount applied by trained individuals is remarkably consistent; what untrained persons apply may vary nearly 20-fold. Most patients tend to apply far too much topical corticosteroid. Show them on a small area of dermatitic or normal skin how to apply a thin film and gently massage it in.

The amounts of topical corticosteroid necessary for four daily applications are shown in Table 1-2. These figures are generous approximations based on precise studies.[4] If the medication is applied only twice daily, halve the numbers. Remember that 30 gm (about one ounce) will suffice for one application to the entire skin of an adult.

Frequency of application

How many times should your patient apply the corticosteroid? The usual advice of three or four daily applications is based on custom rather than reason. With the less potent corticosteroids, applications three or four times a day are probably helpful; with the newer, highly potent fluorinated formulations, one or two applications daily may be enough. On the scalp, one daily application suffices, as the drug usually isn't rubbed off.

There are exceptions. When the emollient effect of the corticosteroid vehicle is desired—as in atopic eczema or irritant (housewife's) hand dermatitis—more frequent applications are desirable. Similarly, if the corticosteroid is likely to be washed off, as in hand dermatitis, as many as 10 to 15 applications a day may be beneficial. Increasing the number of applications is an excellent way to get more effect from hydrocortisone. A flare-up of atopic eczema previously controlled with nightly applications of 1 per cent hydrocortisone may yield to four or five daily applications of the same steroid, and a more potent preparation won't be needed.

Side effects

Systemic

Reassure your patients that topical corticosteroids—unlike systemic corticosteroids—are well tolerated on a long-term basis and seldom produce unde-

TABLE 1-2

Grams of cream or ointment required for four sparing applications for one day

PART	GRAMS (APPROXIMATE)
Face and ears	5
Neck	5
Upper extremity	10
Lower extremity	20
Anterior trunk	15
Posterior trunk	15

Note: 30 gm (approximately one ounce) will suffice for one sparing application to the entire skin of an adult. Because of rounding, the figures above come out to only 25 gm per application.

sirable effects. Surprisingly many patients know of someone whose health was "ruined by steroids" and fear that the same fate awaits them from the tube of corticosteroid cream you've prescribed. Explain to them that while long-term *systemic* corticosteroids invariably produce side effects, long-term *topical* corticosteroids are safe. This reassurance is appropriate for at least 90 per cent of your patients who will be applying corticosteroids only to limited areas. The patient instruction sheet titled "Cortisone Ointments" will reinforce your explanation.

Systemic absorption of a topical corticosteroid does occur; with hydrocortisone approximately 1 per cent of the applied dose is absorbed from noninflamed skin. Corticosteroid absorption increases when skin is inflamed, when high-potency corticosteroids are applied, and when occlusion is used. Infants and children are more susceptible than adults to systemic effects of topical corticosteroids.

In most patients treated with low- and intermediate-strength topical corticosteroids it's impossible to demonstrate any systemic effect. In patients with extensive dermatitis treated with topical corticosteroids, especially if potent or used with occlusion, depression of adrenal cortical function may be demonstrable. This adrenal suppression is usually a laboratory finding without clinical significance; normal adrenal function generally returns less than a week after the drug has been stopped. However, patients undergoing long-term topical corticosteroid treatment of extensive dermatitis should be alerted to the possibility that adrenal suppression may pose a health threat in case of surgery or systemic illness.

Frank adrenal hypercorticism—Cushing's disease—from topical corticosteroids is rare. It occurs occasionally in children whose severe dermatoses require prolonged topical corticosteroids; in these instances it's an unavoidable complication. In treating children with extensive atopic dermatitis, continuing efforts should be made to decrease the strength of the corticosteroid to the minimum required for reasonable control.

Potent corticosteroids should be prescribed only in limited amounts—and then used. Patients are often denied the benefits of topical corticosteroids because of unwarranted fears concerning systemic effects. All too often I encounter children who are miserable with uncontrolled atopic dermatitis because of their parents' unjustified fears of corticosteroid side effects. It's cruel to the child—and the family—to forgo the topical medication. Again, augment your discussion of the safety of topical corticosteroids with the "Cortisone Ointments" patient instruction sheet.

Local side effects

Atrophy

Adverse cutaneous side effects of topical corticosteroids are a more common and more vexing problem than systemic side effects. The ability of potent corticosteroids—especially the newer, fluorinated products—to produce atrophy and acneiform eruptions has not been fully appreciated. In part this is because the changes are gradual and often attributed to the underlying disease rather than the topical drug. Corticosteroids interfere with cellular replication; this effect is minimal with hydrocortisone but may be severe with potent fluorinated corticosteroids. Corticosteroid atrophy is epidermal thinning and wasting of the subcutaneous tissue (see Figure C-32). In skin folds striae may result; in other areas the thinning may cause subcutaneous vessels to be visible. Petechiae and ecchymoses may result. Epidermal thinning of the hands and feet may cause patients to complain of easy fissuring of their fingertips or toes.

In the perianal and genital area, corticosteroid atrophy and the resulting irritation, burning, and redness may be mistaken for uncontrolled dermatitis. Consequently, ever-stronger corticosteroids are used, and the dermatitis is compounded in a vicious cycle. With hydrocortisone there's far less chance of atrophy; it is the drug of choice in treating skin-fold areas, especially genital and perianal. Clinically detectable atrophy from 1 per cent hydrocortisone practically never occurs. With 3 to 5 per cent hydrocortisone preparations low-grade atrophy in skin-fold areas may occur. Using the lowest effective concentration of hydrocortisone in skin-fold areas minimizes the risks of atrophy there.

Rosacealike dermatitis
On the face, potent corticosteroids can cause or aggravate a peculiar acneiform or rosacealike dermatitis (steroid rosacea) (Figures C-39, C-40, and C-41). The picture resembles a combination of dermatitis and acnelike eruption having erythematous scaly patches as well as papules and pustules. When this corticosteroid side effect is superimposed on a preceding dermatitis, such as seborrheic dermatitis, it frequently escapes recognition and gets steadily worse while being treated with a succession of ever-more-potent corticosteroids. Stopping the medication often causes this steroid rosacea to flare up, which further delays the correct diagnosis. Steroid rosacea usually improves with systemic tetracycline; sometimes a short course of systemic corticosteroids is necessary. This rosaceaform corticosteroid complication can be avoided by using only hydrocortisone on the face. The "Cortisone Ointments" patient information sheet stresses the risk of local complications, since these are fairly common.

Rebound dermatitis
Rebound dermatitis may occur when potent corticosteroids are discontinued. This is common in steroid rosacea, where the rosaceaform dermatitis often flares up when the fluorinated corticosteroid is stopped. It's not uncommon in the genital, inguinal, and perianal areas. Resuming the fluorinated corticosteroid only compounds the problem and puts off the moment of truth. Sometimes a two- or three-week course of prednisone is required to suppress rebound dermatitis.

Occlusion

Occlusion greatly potentiates the effect of topical corticosteroids. Occlusion of normal skin increases the penetration of hydrocortisone 10-fold. Occlusion therapy is used mainly for (1) dermatoses of the palms and soles, (2) psoriasis of glabrous skin, (3) any localized patch of severely lichenified dermatitis, and (4) extensive, severe, steroid-responsive dermatitis as an alternative to systemic corticosteroids.

Thin plastic films such as Saran Wrap are useful for occluding small areas. Plastic gloves work well on the hands, plastic bags on the feet, and plastic suits are available for total body occlusion. The trunk can be occluded with a plastic garment bag or plastic trash-can liner with holes cut for arms and head. The occluding plastic is best held in place with a light garment—socks on the feet, a sleeve or thin stocking on the extremities—rather than tape, which may irritate. On skin areas where tape must be used, a relatively non-irritating porous ("paper") product should be employed.

Occlusion should not be used for more than 8 out of 24 hours, as continuously occluded skin may become macerated and dermatitic. As little normal skin should be occluded as possible. It's traditional to use plastic occlusion overnight; this works well for the hands, feet, and similar limited areas. For those requiring total body occlusion with a plastic suit, a shorter three- or four-hour period during waking hours often suffices. The plastic suit is worn next to the skin; the patient may wear ordinary clothing over it. As the patient improves with occlusive therapy it should be gradually withdrawn by using it every other day, later on every third day, to minimize the chance of sudden flare-ups.

CAUTION: **Patients must not exercise while undergoing complete body occlusion with a plastic suit,** since body heat regulation is severely compromised by their inability to evaporate sweat. They should be given written warnings to avoid exercise while wearing the plastic suit.

Since occlusion increases corticosteroid absorption, it also increases the risk of side effects. Systemic corticosteroid effects are generally not a problem when less than 10 per cent of the body is occluded and low- or medium-potency preparations are used. When large areas of the body are occluded, the possibility of systemic corticosteroid side effects must be kept in mind, especially if the drug is highly potent.

The local side effects of occlusion are related mainly to its potentiation of the tendency of strong corticosteroids to produce atrophy. In hot weather miliaria can be a problem. Folliculitis occasionally occurs; then occlusion should be stopped. Occlusion is contraindicated in the presence of pyoderma.

Intralesional corticosteroids

Intralesional corticosteroid injections occupy a position intermediate between topical and systemic therapy. All of the injected intralesional corticosteroid is absorbed. Since it's absorbed slowly, it is usually possible to obtain a local therapeutic effect without measurable systemic effects. When large amounts of corticosteroids are injected intralesionally, systemic effects will be evident.

In intralesional therapy a suspension of slowly soluble corticosteroids is injected into dermatitic skin. Triamcinolone acetonide suspension is the drug of choice; it provides a therapeutic effect lasting 4 to 10 weeks. In the United States, injectable triamcinolone acetonide (Kenalog) is available in concentrations of 10 and 40 mg/ml. The 40 mg/ml concentration, which is intended for intramuscular administration, is not suitable for intralesional injection. For most situations, the undiluted 10 mg/ml suspension is adequate. When using intralesional triamcinolone acetonide for treating acne of the face, however, dilute the suspension to 2 or 3 mg/ml to minimize the chance of atrophy.

Indications for intralesional corticosteroids

Intralesional corticosteroids are most commonly used for relatively small areas of lichenified, stubborn psoriasis, atopic eczema, lichen simplex chronicus, nummular eczema (Figure C-16), and lichen planus. They're also employed in treating alopecia areata. Inflammatory acne lesions are injected with dilute triamcinolone acetonide. Keloids may regress when injected with the undiluted 10 mg/ml suspension, since steroids inhibit fibroblast proliferation. Intralesional injections are used for treating a circumscribed, steroid-responsive lesion requiring corticosteroid penetration into the dermis and subcutis. Extensive dermatoses are not suitable for intralesional treatment, as the large amounts of corticosteroids they require would produce significant systemic side effects.

Technique

Intralesional repository corticosteroids should be injected into the upper subcutis, not intradermally. Intradermal injection—injection with wheal formation—may cause skin atrophy. The proper depth of injection ranges from 3 to 7 mm; with practice one learns to insert the needle with a short, quick jab to penetrate the tough dermis.

A tuberculin syringe with a Luer Lok should be used to attach the needle firmly. Considerable pressure is needed for intralesional injection, and needles attached to an ordinary friction hub tend to become dislodged, with a resultant embarrassing spray of the contents. Long, thin, 1-ml tuberculin-type syringes permit adequate control of the amount of corticosteroid injected. Disposable tuberculin syringes with Luer-Lok hubs have been unobtainable; consequently I still use glass syringes. If you insist on disposables, use the tuberculin syringes with permanently attached 27-gauge needles that are designed for intradermal allergy testing.

The discomfort of injection is minimized by using tiny needles. The best is the 13-mm (half-inch) 30-gauge needle; patients appreciate their thinness. There are brand differences in the sharpness of the disposable 30-gauge needles. The half-inch 30-gauge needles manufactured by MPL Inc. (1820 West Roscoe Street, Chicago, Ill. 60657) are consistently excellent. The bore of the 30-gauge needle is too small to permit withdrawal of the corticosteroid suspension from the vial; for this use a 20- or 22-gauge needle.

Intralesional injections are best performed with a syringe held in one hand (Figure 1-1). After thrusting the needle through the dermis with a short

Topical corticosteroids

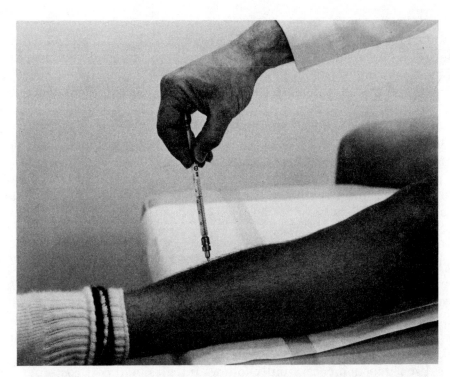

Figure 1-1. Intralesional injection of a corticosteroid into a plaque of psoriasis on a young man's leg. The palm of the hand is squeezed against the plunger to deliver the desired 0.05 to 0.1 ml of suspension to each puncture site. Multiple punctures can be made quickly, since the syringe is gripped in the same way throughout the procedure.

wrist motion, squeeze your palm against the plunger to inject the drug into the subcutis. Note:

1. Use a short wrist-motion jab.
2. Insert the needle perpendicular to the skin surface so it will traverse as little tissue as possible.
3. The depth of injection depends on skin thickness and varies from 3 to 7 mm (one-fourth to one-half the length of a 13-mm needle).
4. Inject 0.05 to 0.1 ml at each puncture. This usually suffices for a 1- to 2-cm^2 area of dermatitis.
5. For lesions larger than 1 to 2 cm^2, space the injection sites approximately 2 cm apart.

Side effects

Systemic

The entire amount of corticosteroid deposited intralesionally is absorbed. Not all corticosteroid withdrawn from a vial is deposited in the tissue; a little drips from the needle between injections and a little flows back out at each puncture site.

Injections of less than 10 mg of triamcinolone acetonide at intervals of more than 90 days are probably free of detectable side effects. With larger

Topical corticosteroids

amounts, systemic effects may occur. After receiving 20 to 30 mg of triamcinolone acetonide intralesionally, it's common for patients with eczema or psoriasis to report improvement in lesions not injected. Triamcinolone acetonide is slowly absorbed from tissue for two to three months; injections at more frequent intervals produce a cumulative effect. No firm rules as to the amount and timing of injections can be given; the systemic effects of intralesional corticosteroids must be kept in mind if more than 10 mg of triamcinolone acetonide are injected every three months.

In performing intralesional injections, you needn't try to prevent an occasional intravascular injection. Systemic side effects from such occasional intravascular injections have not been reported with triamcinolone acetonide suspensions made in the United States.

Local

Atrophy can be troublesome, although it's nearly always temporary. Atrophy usually results either from injecting too superficially (intradermally) or from injecting more than 0.1 ml of corticosteroid at each site. As even temporary atrophy on the face is undesirable, use dilute (2 to 3 mg/ml) triamcinolone acetonide on the face.

Localized infection occasionally follows intralesional corticosteroid injections of the hands or feet but practically never occurs elsewhere. Its extreme recalcitrance makes me reluctant to inject the hands or feet. The repository corticosteroid interferes with the inflammatory and repair processes, and patients developing such infections may require multiple incisions and drainage procedures in addition to weeks of systemic antibiotics.

Putting it together

The following examples will illustrate how to employ topical corticosteroids optimally.

1. **Patient:** A 7-year-old girl with dry, scaling patches of low-grade atopic eczema on the face.

   Treatment: One per cent hydrocortisone cream applied thinly four times a day. White petrolatum applied after the hydrocortisone at bedtime, and during the day as desired if the skin is too dry.

   Rationale: Fluorinated steroids should be avoided in treating the face. As the dermatitis is mild, you choose 1 per cent hydrocortisone rather than a higher concentration. An ointment is usually more effective for dry dermatitis, but is less cosmetically acceptable than a cream. Compromise by using a cream and have the patient follow it at bedtime with petrolatum to provide an ointment effect. The four-times-a-day application is desirable for its emollient action as well as its anti-inflammatory effect.

2. **Patient:** A 10-year-old boy with moderately severe dry, fissured atopic eczema of the antecubitals, popliteals, and backs of the hands.

   Treatment: Triamcinolone acetonide 0.025 per cent, both cream and ointment. Have the patient use the cream on one side, the ointment on the other, and see which is more beneficial. Application three or four times a day usually suffices for the antecubitals and popliteals. The hands should receive more frequent applications.

Rationale: An intermediate-strength corticosteroid generally suffices in this situation. While ointments usually are better than creams for chronic atopic eczema, some patients don't tolerate them. The patient has the final word. Hand dermatitis is stubborn. It requires frequent applications for the vehicles to achieve their emollient effects.

3. **Patient:** A 46-year-old man whose chronic seborrheic dermatitis of the glabella, forehead, nasolabial folds, scalp edges, and ears is itchy.

Treatment: For the face, 2 to 3 per cent hydrocortisone cream applied thinly at bedtime and massaged in well. Tell the patient that if he isn't better in a week, he should apply it twice daily. If the eyebrows are involved, the cream should be applied with a moist finger to convert it to a liquid for better skin delivery. For the scalp edges and ears a fluorinated corticosteroid gel, lotion, or solution applied sparingly at bedtime.

Rationale: Using 2 to 3 per cent hydrocortisone, rather than the traditional 1 per cent, will result in a faster initial response and require less frequent applications for long-term suppression. While hydrocortisone could be used for the scalp edges and ears, these sites respond less well to corticosteroids than the face; a fluorinated corticosteroid is preferable and usually safe in these areas. Once-daily applications to scalp edges and ears generally suffice; bedtime is a convenient and specific treatment time.

4. **Patient:** A 56-year-old woman who has had a patch of chronic, itching, lichenified dermatitis of the occipital scalp and nape of the neck for over 10 years. A previous physician prescribed 1 per cent hydrocortisone lotion; another gave her 0.1 per cent triamcinolone acetonide cream; neither topical controlled her dermatitis. You diagnose lichen simplex chronicus.

Treatment: A potent fluorinated corticosteroid in liquid, gel, or solution form applied twice daily. Ask the patient to return in two to three weeks; if the eruption doesn't improve dramatically, inject 10 mg/ml of triamcinolone acetonide intralesionally.

Rationale: Chronic lichenified dermatitis tends to resist corticosteroids; this patient requires a potent drug and a vehicle that delivers it to the scalp. One physician had used the right vehicle but the wrong steroid; the other, the reverse. Always inquire as to previous topical corticosteroid therapy; it may enable you to repeat previous successes and avoid failure. If a lichenified chronic dermatitis fails to respond to a potent corticosteroid, it's either because of inadequate penetration or because the process is not corticosteroid-sensitive. Intralesional injection penetrates the thickened skin.

References

1. Maibach HI, Stoughton RB: Topical corticosteroids. *Med Clin N Amer* 57:1253, 1973

2. Sneddon IB: Clinical use of topical corticosteroids. *Drugs* 11:193, 1973

3. Robertson DB, Maibach HI: Topical corticosteroids. *Int J Dermatol* 21:59, 1982

4. Schlagel CA, Sanborn EC: The weights of topical preparations required for total and partial body inunction. *J Invest Dermatol* 42:253, 1964

Diagnosing dermatitis 2

Diagnosing dermatitis is often difficult for the experienced dermatologist. No wonder the generalist may be frustrated when trying to match the patient's rash with such terms as nummular eczema, dyshidrotic eczema, dermatitis venenata, atopic eczema, asteatotic eczema, ad (almost) infinitum. This chapter describes a simplified way of diagnosing dermatitis that bypasses many traditional diagnostic labels. A simple—and therapeutically more useful—approach to diagnosing dermatitis recognizes that all dermatoses result from the often complex interaction between exogenous and endogenous factors.

Dermatitis—a useful concept

Dermatitis and eczema are interchangeable terms describing skin disorders that are characterized by superficial scaling, erythema, papules, and vesiculation. Usually *dermatitis* and *eczema* are applied to disorders whose cause is unknown. In general, if the rash is known to have a specific etiology it is not referred to as dermatitis but is classified in terms of the cause. Thus a fungal infection of the feet, although it looks like dermatitis, is diagnosed as tinea pedis. The term *dermatitis* thus is used in both a specific way and also in a general sense.

Dermatitis in its more specific sense describes clinical entities having skin eruptions that fit the broad morphologic definition of dermatitis. Atopic dermatitis, seborrheic dermatitis, and psoriasis are all dermatoses. They are well-delineated, genetically determined skin dysfunctions. *Dermatitis* is also used as a general term to describe any eczematous rash of unknown etiology that can't be classified among the major genetically determined dermatoses; i.e., atopic dermatitis, psoriasis, and seborrheic dermatitis. Unfortunately, most dermatoses encountered by the physician cannot be classified into these three major groupings. Since dermatology began as a morphologic specialty, it was natural for physicians to attempt to classify the mass of dermatoses into morphologic entities. Unfortunately, the resulting welter of terminology has led only to the illusion of knowledge.

Those confusing terms

Why disregard much of the complex terminology attached to dermatitis? Because it's largely useless in understanding what's actually going on.

The meaninglessness of much of the terminology becomes clear when one sees patients with chronic dermatitis. They've often been given a variety of diagnostic labels by several capable, experienced dermatologists. For example, one of my patients with hand dermatitis had previously been examined by three competent dermatologists and received three different morphologic diagnoses! Initially the eruption was mild and diagnosed as irritant (housewife's) hand dermatitis. When it got worse and took the form of round, somewhat infiltrated eczematous patches, the next specialist diagnosed nummular eczema. Failing to get relief, the patient consulted a third expert, who diagnosed psoriasis of the hands. When she got to me, she had typical psoriasis of the elbows and scalp; dermatologist number three was correct.

This woman didn't have three different skin disorders; she had psoriasis all along. However, in the early stages it wasn't morphologically typical and therefore couldn't be diagnosed. Wouldn't it have been simpler to be content with the label *dermatitis* until the nature of the process became clear?

No one denies the value of morphologic classifications when possible. It's both prognostically and therapeutically useful to distinguish seborrheic dermatitis from scalp psoriasis. The management and prognosis of irritant hand dermatitis differ markedly from those of psoriasis of the hands. What I am stressing is that morphology often fails to provide a rational classification; sometimes it misleads. Rather than struggle with fuzzy terminology, we can look in a different way at the many ill-defined dermatoses we encounter.

Exogenous and endogenous factors in dermatitis

Dermatitis results from the interaction of endogenous and exogenous factors. Analyzing a patient's dermatitis from this aspect lets you understand the processes responsible for the disorder.

Endogenous refers to the skin itself malfunctioning. The mechanism is usually unknown; the dysfunction is genetically determined. Psoriasis, atopic dermatitis, and seborrheic dermatitis are clinically defined disorders that in their "textbook" form are entirely endogenous. They are prone to spontaneous worsening and remission; these changes frustrate clinicians, since one can never be sure whether they're part of the disease process or caused by external factors. While endogenous factors are usually genetically determined and idiopathic, there is an exception: Stasis dermatitis results from defective circulation, usually to the legs.

Exogenous describes the external factors influencing dermatitis. These can be classified as irritants and allergens. Irritants chemically damage skin. Soap, detergents, solvents, and abrasive cleansers are among the many commonly encountered irritants. Persons vary greatly in their response to irritants. Allergens act by an acquired immunologic mechanism. In North America, poison ivy and poison oak are the most common causes of "pure" allergic contact dermatitis. Sunlight and humidity are other exogenous factors that can affect dermatitis.

The melange

Most dermatoses result from a combination of endogenous and exogenous factors. Atopic dermatitis is frequently aggravated by overuse of soap (an irritant) and application of irritating over-the-counter topical remedies. Allergic contact dermatitis caused by a topical medicament may complicate any dermatitis but is especially frequent in stasis dermatitis. It's the clinician's task to sort out the various factors as a preliminary to rational management. Here are some guidelines.

Finding endogenous factors

The directed history is critical. Suspect endogenous factors when there is a long history of dermatitis, especially with intermittent clearing. Did the patient have dermatitis in childhood? Next inquire as to atopic dermatitis, psoriasis, or any type of chronic skin condition in close blood relatives. If a young woman with patchy hand dermatitis tells you her mother had hand eczema, you can be fairly sure her dermatitis is basically endogenous.

Examine the entire skin. Dermatitis of the antecubitals and popliteals is evidence of atopic eczema. Don't neglect the perianal skin; a sharply demarcated eruption of the gluteal cleft suggests psoriasis. Pitting of the nails, dermatitis of the glans penis, and chronic scaling of ear canals all point to psoriasis—mild forms of which are common. Examine the entire skin even if the patient protests that it's normal. Patients are often embarrassed by, or unaware of, rashes elsewhere. Tell patients reluctant to have their "normal" skins examined, "I want to examine your normal skin as it will help me treat your rash." Figures C-33, C-34, and C-35 illustrate the diagnostic value of examining a patient's entire skin.

Detecting exogenous factors

The type of history will depend on the rash's distribution; do your detailed questioning after examining the patient. A patient with hand dermatitis requires a totally different history from one with foot dermatitis. Only a few of the many agents that might cause hand dermatitis could conceivably play a role in foot dermatitis. Taking a suitable exposure history is a challenging art; here are a few guidelines.

Topical applications are some of the most common exogenous causes of dermatitis. Get a history of all topical applications the patient has used— creams, ointments, antibiotics, antiseptics, cosmetics, sun protectives, and so on. Details of over-the-counter preparations and prescription items are necessary. Patients' memories are often unreliable; have them bring in everything they have used on their rashes.

Find out if there is any relationship to vacation, hobbies, trips, sun exposure, or work. Be reluctant to diagnose an industrial cause, for it has serious social and medical consequences. In my experience, the diagnosis of industrial dermatitis is often incorrectly applied.

Irritants

Irritants are some of the most common exogenous causes of dermatitis. The diagnosis of irritant factors is circumstantial and unsatisfactory. We're all exposed to such irritants as soap and detergents; we don't all have dermatitis. On the other hand, any dermatitis will be aggravated by exposure to irritants. We lack a test to confirm the diagnosis of irritant dermatitis. A high degree of suspicion leads to elimination of possible offenders. Improvement suggests that irritants were responsible—but one can't be certain, since topical corticosteroids are almost invariably simultaneously employed.

While it's universally recognized that soap, solvents, paint, and abrasive cleansers are irritants, it is not appreciated that often substances designed for skin application are low-grade irritants. Many cosmetics, skin lubricants, antiseptic creams, and even topical corticosteroids are low-grade irritants. When used repeatedly, they can cause or aggravate dermatitis in a susceptible individual. Irritant dermatitis from preparations designed to improve skin is often overlooked. Irritation from cosmetics is a common cause of facial dermatitis in women. Remember that there's enormous individual variation in sensitivity to irritants.

Dry air can irritate by reducing skin moisture. The nonspecific dermatitis labeled asteatotic is common during winter in cold climates, since the low humidity reduces the skin's water content. While most irritants are chemicals, sunlight can produce "toxic" or irritant dermatitis. Sunlight may also produce allergic dermatitis.

Allergens

Poison ivy and poison oak are common causes of allergic contact dermatitis in North America. Topical medicaments are the next most frequent. Allergy to nickel is common in women, infrequent in men. Cosmetics (especially perfumes), rubber, and epoxy glues are at the top of the almost endless list of known sensitizers.

Fortunately we can test for contact allergy with the patch test. Scratch and intradermal tests are useless.* The patch test is simple in theory but tricky in execution. Leave it to the experts.

Allergens, while a less common cause of dermatitis than endogenous or irritant factors, must be thoroughly searched for. The reward of uncovering a causative allergen is cure. Avoiding further allergen contact cures allergic contact dermatitis. Allergic contact dermatitis is a complex subject; Cronin's excellent text[1] and Hjorth and Fregert's chapter[2] provide a wealth of details.

---

*An exception is contact urticaria, in which whealing occurs 20 to 30 minutes after contact.

Synthesis

In diagnosing dermatitis the history, morphology, and distribution of the rash must all be considered in elucidating the role of endogenous and exogenous factors. Sometimes, as in typical psoriasis or atopic eczema, the task is easy. Often it is not. Hand dermatitis presents a formidable diagnostic challenge since it's usually multifactorial and lesion morphology is often nondescript. A practical, step-by-step approach to diagnosing hand dermatitis is given in the hand dermatitis unit.

Uncertainties

Diagnosing dermatitis depends on excluding specific causes. As in any other diagnosis based on exclusion, e.g., essential hypertension, there always remains the nagging doubt: Was something overlooked? Even experts occasionally fall into these traps:

1. A fungal infection mimics another disease. Tinea corporis can perfectly simulate nummular eczema. Dermatophyte infection of the hands often looks just like psoriasis. Do a KOH exam (see Appendix).
2. Scabies can produce eczematous changes and be mistaken for dermatitis—especially on the hands. Think of scabies with any intensely itching rash; examine the entire skin for burrows.
3. Bowen's disease (intraepidermal squamous-cell carcinoma) often presents as a recalcitrant, localized patch of dermatitis. A biopsy will settle the issue. Biopsying any persistent dermatitis is a good idea. Occasionally a specific diagnosis, such as lichen planus, will result.
4. Drug eruptions are occasionally eczematous. The localized fixed drug eruption may mislead the unsuspecting.
5. Photosensitivity can mimic an airborne contact dermatitis as well as endogenous dermatitis.
6. The patient has two disorders. For example, in men psoriasis of the groin may coexist with tinea cruris.
7. The overlooked allergen or irritant is the most common error. There are legions of possible contactants. Allergy to a preservative widely used in ointment bases occasionally maintains a dermatitis while the physician switches from one topical to another. What physician considers the wife's perfume when diagnosing arm dermatitis in a man? Or rubber in eyelash curlers as causing eyelid dermatitis? Persistence, skill, and luck ferreted these out.

When a dermatitis fails to improve, question your patient repeatedly about what he's applying to his skin. Patients "sneak" cosmetics, or consider the use of a hand lotion too inconsequential to mention.

Doctor, what's causing my rash?

Physicians dread this question when dealing with dermatitis. People like simple, clear-cut answers. They want to know the cause so they can eliminate it and be cured. They're most unhappy when told it's a matter of multiple factors—one of them being endogenous.

An explanation of irritants and allergens is well accepted, but the concept of endogenous factors is troublesome. I tell patients that their skin is "misbehaving" and that this results from a "built-in" skin defect. It helps to point out that other ailments such as arthritis, high blood pressure, and diabetes are results of the body's malfunctioning.

A family history of endogenous dermatitis makes your task easier; point out that defective skin "runs" in their family. Patients with psoriasis will often accept the implications—a fringe benefit of advertisements for remedies to heal the "heartbreak" of psoriasis.

Stress the positive. Emphasize that while the underlying cause of the endogenous dermatitis remains unknown, the rash can usually be controlled and often be cleared up. The authority of the written word helps. Be sure the patient receives and reads the appropriate information sheet. In spite of your best efforts some patients will be dissatisfied. They will keep trying to blame their chronic dermatoses on pollution, diet, or nerves. Many will shift from physician to physician in a never-ending search for a cure.

Neurodermatitis and other nonsense

It isn't only patients who have trouble accepting the concept of endogenous skin dysfunction. Physicians have the same problem. For centuries toxins and dietary problems were blamed for skin disorders. Bleeding as a method of ridding the body of toxins has long been abandoned, but purging as a treatment for skin diseases was fashionable well into this century. Fortunately, these methods have been discarded. Unfortunately, one delusion persists: that "nerves" cause dermatitis. The erroneous notion of psychogenic dermatitis is maintained in the term *neurodermatitis*.

The word *neurodermatitis* was coined by 19th-century physicians who believed that certain dermatoses resulted from dysfunction of cutaneous nerves—in other words, a neuritis. The term persisted even after it became clear that cutaneous nerves do not cause dermatitis. However, its meaning was changed. Now *neurodermatitis* is applied to the notion that certain chronic dermatoses represent a neurosis, i.e., a psychological disorder. Yet there's no evidence that psychogenic disorders cause dermatitis, and a good deal of evidence that they do not. *Neurodermatitis* is a misleading, 19th-century label that should be expelled from our vocabulary.

That the nervous system can influence skin disorders is undeniable. Emotional upsets and nervous stress may aggravate psoriasis, atopic dermatitis, and other skin disorders just as they may aggravate hypertension, arthritis, and diabetes. Yet no one maintains the latter are psychogenic in origin! Not infrequently, one encounters patients who blame themselves for their psoriasis or eczema since they have been told it's caused by nervousness. Putting the responsibility for such disorders on the patient's back is not only cruel, it's medically erroneous and therapeutically sterile.

Treatment

This chapter covers general principles of diagnosis; treatment is described in the disease units on psoriasis, atopic dermatitis, seborrheic dermatitis, and hand dermatitis. When patients' symptoms don't fit the standard clinical entities, match your treatment to the disorders they most closely resemble. A catch-all unit on dermatitis is included. The physician section discusses the treatment of dermatitis, while the patient version provides treatment advice and a diagnostic label. Use this information sheet for the many patients whose dermatitis doesn't fit the traditional major categories of dermatoses. Since you will treat most dermatoses with topical corticosteroids, use the "Cortisone Ointments" information sheet to improve patients' understanding and compliance.

References

1. Cronin E: *Contact Dermatitis*. Edinburgh: Churchill Livingstone, 1980

2. Hjorth N, Fregert S: Contact dermatitis. In *Textbook of Dermatology* (Rook A, Wilkinson DS, Ebling FJG, eds), 3rd ed, p 363. Oxford: Blackwell, 1979

Dermatologic surgery

3

Skin lesions that involve only the epidermis can frequently be cured by superficial skin surgery that takes only a few minutes and yields good cosmetic results. These techniques, although simple, are scarcely mentioned in surgical texts. This chapter describes easily mastered techniques for removal of superficial skin lesions. When lesions involve the dermis, conventional full-thickness skin excision is usually best. Full-thickness skin excision is the treatment of choice for most skin cancers, since it gives superior cosmetic results with the advantage of histologic control of the margins of the lesions. Full-thickness skin surgery is well described in two recently published manuals.[1,2] This chapter discusses only some special techniques.

The tools

Curette

The curette is a scraping instrument; its German name means sharp spoon. The curette used by bone surgeons and some dermatologists does indeed have a spoonlike shape; however, most dermatologists in the United States use the hollow-ring curette (Figures 3-1 and 3-2). The ring curette affords superior visibility and control in treating lesions. The opening of the ring curette may be either round or oval; the round is easier to sharpen. Curettes are available in many sizes; I use a 5-mm curette (diameter of the cutting ring) as a basic tool and a 2-mm curette for small lesions. Ring curettes are available from surgical-supply houses specializing in dermatologic instruments, such as Robbins Instruments, Inc. (2 North Passaic Avenue, Chatham, N.J. 07929) and George Tiemann and Company (21-28 45th Road, Long Island City, N.Y. 11101).

Curettes must be kept sharp. They will dull rapidly if allowed to rattle against other instruments in a pack or tray, so cover their ends with tubing (Figure 3-1). Most rubber and plastic tubing disintegrates with autoclaving. Silastic tubing (Dow), available from laboratory-equipment suppliers, does not. While surgical firms resharpen curettes, you can do it quickly with a special tapering tubular whetstone available from surgical suppliers.

The chalazion curette

This curette, borrowed from our ophthalmologic colleagues, is a small, cup-shaped curette with a long, narrow stem. It's sized according to the diameter of the cup (Figures 3-1 and 3-2). The chalazion curette is a useful instrument for shelling out milia and small cysts; the larger sizes are helpful in scraping the walls of inflamed cysts. You can't sharpen these curettes, so guard their ends with protective tubing.

Serrated iris scissors

Protuberant benign skin lesions are often dealt with by snipping them off flush with the surrounding skin. Skin tags, pedunculated nevi (Figures C-23 and C-24), and protuberant keratoses are among lesions eminently suitable for scissors removal. The ordinary curved iris scissors—no matter how sharp—tends to slip when cutting the tough epidermis. Having one blade serrated prevents slippage and vastly improves the usefulness of iris scissors in skin surgery. Serrating one blade is done to order by specialized surgical suppliers. Either blade may be serrated.

Comedo extractor

The comedo extractor puts circumferential pressure on a comedo or milium to "pop" it out. There are many designs; the wire-loop Schamberg model (Figures 3-1 and 3-2) is popular.

Punch

The punch, designed for removing the full thickness of the skin, is not an instrument of superficial skin surgery. The smaller sizes are useful for rapid skin biopsies. Various sizes can be used to remove a round lesion precisely.

Punches with small knurled handles that are rotated by twisting between the fingers are superior to the older, large-handled Keyes punch. Punches are available in 0.5-mm gradations from 1 to 10 mm in diameter. The smallest I use is 1.5 mm in diameter; the largest, 10. The most useful sizes are from 1.5 to 5 mm; it's helpful to have these in 0.5-mm increments. Above the 5-mm size, 1-mm gradations suffice. Punches must be kept sharp. Ends should be covered with tubing to protect their edges during sterilization. They can be sharpened with a tapered, round whetstone.

Forceps

Splinter forceps and jewelers' forceps (available from surgical suppliers) are inexpensive surgical tools. Both have tapering, pointed ends; a splinter for-

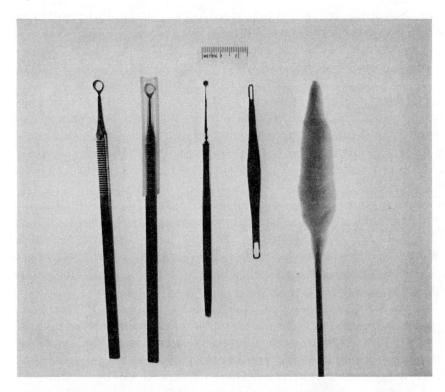

Figure 3-1. From left to right: Orentreich ring curette, curette protected with Silastic tubing, chalazion curette, Schamberg comedo extractor, and homemade liquid nitrogen applicator.

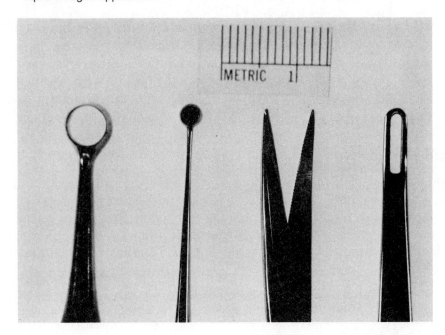

Figure 3-2. Closeup views, from left to right, of Orentreich ring curette, chalazion curette, curved iris scissors with one serrated blade, and Schamberg comedo extractor.

Dermatologic surgery

ceps has serrated tips, which are ideal for removing sutures. The smooth jewelers' forceps is used for gently manipulating tiny bits of tissue and removing the smallest of foreign bodies.

Hemostatics

Control of bleeding after superficial skin surgery may be accomplished with (1) pressure and time, (2) noncaustic packing such as gelatin foam or oxidized cellulose, (3) chemical styptics such as ferric chloride, Monsel's solution, aluminum chloride, and trichloroacetic acid, or (4) electrocoagulation of the wound base.

Chemical styptics are protein precipitants that cause significant cellular damage. Electrodesiccation thermally destroys protein and cells. Electrodesiccation of the wound base is the most scarring hemostatic technique and should be avoided whenever possible. This stricture against electrodesiccation of entire wounds does not apply to point electrocoagulation of bleeding vessels during excisional surgery.

Of the chemical styptics, I prefer to use ferric iron in the form of either Monsel's solution (ferric subsulfate) or ferric chloride tincture. Unlike trichloroacetic acid, ferric iron doesn't damage intact skin. Monsel's solution is commercially available; ferric chloride tincture is easily prepared.*

Chemical styptics should be used only on superficial intradermal wounds. Full-thickness defects exposing subcutaneous fat are not suitable terrain for ferric iron or other chemical styptics. Hemostasis after full-thickness skin removal can be accomplished by suturing, point electrodesiccation of bleeding vessels, pressure, or packing with an inert hemostatic.

Gentlest—and least scarring—of all hemostatics are inert materials such as gelatin foam and oxidized cellulose. I use 7-mm-thick gelatin foam (Gelfoam) packaged as 20- by 60-mm strips in individual sterile envelopes. Since only a small part of a packet is needed, I tear off a portion with sterile forceps and save the remainder in the envelope. Although this economy breaches absolute sterility, it doesn't matter in skin surgery.

Liquid nitrogen

Liquid nitrogen is ideal for removing warts and benign superficial keratoses since, when used lightly on superficial lesions, it produces less scarring than other destructive techniques.† It can be applied with a large cotton-wool swab (dipstick) or sprayed on. For superficial lesions, I prefer the dipstick (Figure 3-1) technique. Dip a large, cotton-tipped applicator into liquid nitro-

---

*To a one-pound (450-gm) jar of reagent-grade ferric chloride add 150 ml of water. Shake occasionally over the next two days. Then slowly add 80 ml of 95 to 99 per cent isopropyl alcohol. CAUTION: **Considerable heat is produced.** The alcohol serves as a bacteriostat. After thorough mixing, let stand several hours for the sediment to settle (no need to filter) and pour into small, dark bottles for use in minor surgery.

†Liquid nitrogen destruction should be limited to clearly benign lesions. If the nature of the lesion is in doubt, use cold-steel surgery to provide a specimen for histology.

gen and apply it to the lesion. Use either large manufactured cotton- or rayon-wool-tipped applicators (such as used for proctoscopy) or homemade applicators. I use the commercial ones as disposables for treating anal, genital, or other potentially contaminated lesions. The large commercial swabs, while blunt-ended, are readily shaped to a point.

Homemade applicators are superior. Start with a thin wooden rod about 25 cm long and, ideally, one-eighth inch (3 mm) in diameter. This doweling is obtainable from lumberyards or hobby shops. Apply an adhesive material such as Hollister medical adhesive* or spirit gum. Tightly wind a small amount of cotton wool onto the stick. Add layers of cotton wool—and light applications of adhesive material—until you produce a large, tapered applicator like the one shown in Figure 3-1.

Liquid nitrogen is available in most larger cities. Liquid nitrogen suppliers provide large steel vacuum drums (Dewar flasks) in sizes holding 20, 30, 40, or more liters. A simple valve permits removal of small quantities, which are conveniently held in ordinary Thermos bottles or small vacuum-walled containers sold for this purpose. CAUTION: **Liquid nitrogen containers must never be tightly stoppered; they will explode.** Drill holes in the stoppers of Thermos bottles. At the end of the day, return unused liquid nitrogen to the large storage flask. I use a 20-liter tank; it needs refilling every three weeks.

Tape

The newer, acrylic-based tapes are nonallergenic and rarely irritating. Gentlest are the "paper" and other highly permeable tapes. At least one brand, Micropore (3M Company), is available in a flesh color, which patients may prefer to the traditional white. Acrylic tapes made of fabric (Dermicel) are more durable and may adhere better than "paper" tape. Like "paper" tapes, fabric tapes are permeable (nonocclusive) and don't macerate the underlying skin. There is no reason to use older kinds of tape for skin wounds.

Using tape to support wounds after excisional surgery permits early suture removal and minimizes wound dehiscence. I use nonsterile, flesh-colored tape. To make the tape stick firmly to the skin, paint spirit gum on the skin before applying the tape. Hollister medical adhesive spray is an alternative adhesive, but less convenient. Wound support in hairy areas is a problem because the growing hair soon loosens the tape. Flexible collodion is an alternative to tape; unfortunately, it usually lasts no more than a day or two. It will stick longer if spirit gum or Hollister medical adhesive spray is applied first.

Adhesives

Tincture of benzoin is often painted on patients' skin to make tape stick, but it occasionally causes a nasty dermatitis. Far better is spirit gum, a resin-

---

*Dow Corning medical adhesive B, manufactured for Hollister, Inc., 211 East Chicago Avenue, Chicago, Ill. 60611. In the United States it's distributed through pharmacies (not surgical suppliers) for use by "ostomy" patients to seal bags and appliances to their skin.

based adhesive that actors use to affix wigs and mustaches. It's available from companies that sell theatrical cosmetics. It is cheap, and its high alcohol content assures sterility. If evaporation thickens it excessively, thin it with isopropyl alcohol or alcohol mixed with a little acetone. Allergy to spirit gum is rare.

Spirit gum has another advantage: It's waterproof. Tape applied over it will stick in spite of getting wet. Patients are pleased that they can shower and bathe—but caution them not to rub or scrub the tape. Remnants of spirit gum can be removed with acetone or nail-polish remover.

Even stickier and longer lasting than spirit gum is Hollister medical adhesive, a nonsensitizing aerosol silicone. It's sprayed onto the skin and allowed to dry for a minute before the tape is applied. Hollister medical adhesive is insoluble in water, and "paper" or fabric tape applied over it will usually stick to nonhairy skin for one to two weeks even if repeatedly wetted. Since Hollister adhesive is sprayed on, it's awkward to use on the face, and precise application to small areas is not possible. After applying the tape, dust a bland dusting powder onto the surrounding skin, as otherwise the remaining adhesive will cling tenaciously to clothing. Excess adhesive can be removed with acetone. Tell patients they can remove any excess adhesive with nail-polish remover. Since the spray nozzle tends to clog, wipe the spray tip with a cotton swab moistened with acetone after spraying.

Electrosurgery

Electrosurgical* techniques are popular for destroying tissue. The types of currents produced and their actions vary; they all depend on the production of heat. In my opinion, electrosurgical destruction has two applications: (1) point electrocoagulation of bleeding vessels during surgery and (2) destroying small telangiectases such as vascular spiders. In destroying small blood vessels, bipolar current is superior to monopolar, and pinpoint epilating needles should be used.

A brief diatribe against electrodesiccation
Electrodesiccation (electrocoagulation) of skin lesions is fast and simple. Why do I believe it should be abandoned?

1. Other techniques cause less scarring. Burn scars are uniquely severe and unsightly. Why deliberately produce a burn scar by electrodesiccation? Liquid nitrogen, curettage, scissors removal, and scalpel surgery all produce superior cosmetic results with equivalent amounts of tissue destruction.
2. It's a "blind" procedure. With curettage, scissors removal, and scalpel surgery one feels and sees the depth of destruction and removal. Not so with electrodesiccation. Liquid nitrogen destruction has the same handicap.

---

*Electrodesiccation and electrocoagulation are techniques of tissue destruction using high-frequency electric currents. The electrical energy is converted to heat; these methods burn tissue. Electrodesiccation usually means superficial destruction with a monopolar current, while electrocoagulation refers to the use of a bipolar current to produce a deeper effect.

Dermatologic surgery

3. In thermally "cooking" the tissue, electrodesiccation prevents histologic examination. Curettage, scissors removal, and other cold-steel techniques provide a specimen for histologic confirmation of the diagnosis. The margins of deeper lesions excised with punch or scalpel can be studied for completeness of removal. Again, liquid nitrogen suffers from this same drawback.

Since electrodesiccation suffers from all these handicaps and provides no medical advantage, I have abandoned it except for the two techniques mentioned earlier. Electrodestruction of benign lesions is traditional and popular; unfortunately it's an inferior technique that should be abandoned by critical physicians seeking the best results.

Techniques

Curettage

Curettage is best performed using local anesthesia, although some physicians treat multiple superficial keratoses without anesthesia. For keratoses and superficial warts, the curette is held like a pencil in one hand; with short, swift movements, the lesion is scraped from the skin. The fingers of the other hand should stretch the skin tightly during curettage. When warts and deeper lesions are shelled out, it helps to incise the rim first with a pointed, curved scissors to penetrate the epidermis. Next the curette is used to find the cleavage plane between wart and skin and scoop the lesion out.

After curettage, hemostasis can be instantly achieved with ferric chloride tincture or Monsel's solution. If cosmetic considerations are paramount, use pressure with gauze moistened with a little local anesthetic-epinephrine mixture, or pack with gelatin foam.

Not only does curettage provide tissue for histology, but the feel of lesions during curettage is helpful in diagnosis. Basal-cell carcinomas, for example, have a mushy consistency. Histologic examination of tissue fragments obtained by curettage is simplified when they're allowed to clot together before formalin fixation. Remove bloody fragments from the curette with the point of a scissors or a wooden stick and place them on a piece of smooth paper or on the inside of the specimen bottle, above the formalin. After 5 to 10 minutes immerse the tissue clot in the fixative. Result: a single, easily processed specimen.

Using the comedo extractor

The comedo extractor permits rapid, simple removal of milia (whiteheads) and similar small superficial cysts. After a tiny nick is made in the overlying skin, firm pressure is applied, with the lesion midway in the extractor's loop. Further emptying action is exerted by sliding the extractor's end toward the lesion while maintaining pressure. CAUTION: **Extractors may slip!** When working near the eyes, direct the instrument's pressure away from them and shield the eyes with one hand.

Liquid nitrogen

In using the simple dipstick technique, dip your large, cotton-tipped applicator (Figure 3-1) in the Thermos of liquid nitrogen and apply its tip to the lesion. As liquid nitrogen runs down the applicator, the skin at the tip turns white; this ice front gradually spreads outward. Stop when the visible freezing extends just beyond the lesion. For a 5- to 10-mm-diameter lesion, 10 to 20 seconds of liquid nitrogen application are generally enough.

Larger and deeper lesions take longer. Lesions over 15 mm in diameter are best treated by moving the applicator about so as to freeze the entire area without freezing too deeply.

The duration of freezing also depends on the speed of delivery of liquid nitrogen from your applicator. A large, completely saturated applicator will freeze lesions more rapidly than a small, drier one. Aim to achieve a steady release of small droplets onto the lesion. If large droplets run over the surrounding skin, you have too much liquid nitrogen on your applicator; flick off the excess with a snap of your wrist. The rate of delivery of liquid nitrogen can be adjusted by altering the applicator's angle; the closer to vertical, the more rapid the flow of liquid nitrogen.

Applying liquid nitrogen is an art that can be learned only by doing. If in doubt, err by underfreezing. It's simple to treat residuals a second time; scars from excessive freezing are another matter. Be suspicious of any lesion that doesn't respond to liquid nitrogen. If in doubt, biopsy.

This simple applicator technique has been abandoned by some dermatologists in favor of direct spraying of liquid nitrogen onto the lesion. The spray technique is more difficult and requires specialized equipment. Its chief value lies in the treatment of malignancies, as it can freeze more deeply than the applicator technique. Since I prefer to excise malignant lesions surgically, I haven't used the spray technique.

Punch biopsy

When biopsying, mark the area to be biopsied before injecting the local anesthetic. After anesthesia—and punch biopsy should always be done with anesthesia—immobilize the skin with the fingers of one hand while coring out a cylinder of skin by twirling the punch between the fingers of the other. As the punch traverses from the dermis into the fat, resistance lessens. You are now deep enough. When the punch is removed, the core of tissue usually pops up slightly and can be snipped off at the level of the subcutaneous fat with a curved iris scissors without using a forceps. Because forceps may squeeze and distort small punch-biopsy specimens, it's preferable to hold specimens with a small hypodermic needle.

Hemostasis after punch biopsy can be accomplished with gelatin foam packing. Defects from 1.5- and 2.0-mm punches usually don't require suturing and will heal virtually invisibly. Punch defects in the 2- to 3.5-mm range can generally be closed completely with a single suture. Complete closure of larger punch defects frequently leads to dog-earing and should be avoided. Partial closure of a round defect is practical and is discussed in the next section.

With a 1.5-mm punch you can take biopsy specimens in cosmetically sensitive areas with virtually perfect results. It's better cosmetically to take two or three 1.5-mm samples from a large lesion than one 3- or 4-mm chunk. When several small specimens are taken from a single lesion, they can be combined in one tissue bottle and the pathologist informed that they can be mounted on the same slide.

Multiple small biopsies are an excellent way to delineate the extent of a basal-cell carcinoma with indistinct borders. The location of each biopsy should be sketched out and each specimen submitted in a separate bottle.

The punch is an effective tool for removing small, round lesions. The margins of the lesion should be marked prior to infiltrating the local anesthetic. After the anesthetic has been infiltrated the diameter of the lesion is measured, the punch chosen, and the lesion removed. This fast method produces excellent results with small lesions.

Excision with partial closure

Concern about closing wounds makes some physicians reluctant to excise lesions in locations where the traditional excision and complete closure are not feasible. While complete closure is desirable, it's by no means necessary. Wounds left open often heal with excellent cosmetic results, especially on the face. Simple excision and allowing the wound to granulate are effective in areas such as the nose, where complete closure would require grafting or other plastic surgical procedures. In these situations, my preference is to close the wound partially with sutures, being careful not to distort the tissues. The unclosed portion is allowed to heal secondarily. I have described the technique in detail elsewhere.[3] It permits the physician with limited surgical skills to utilize the advantages of excisional surgery in areas where the conventional fusiform excision and complete closure aren't possible. A minimum amount of normal tissue is sacrificed, and the tissues aren't compromised if further surgical procedures are needed.

If excision with partial closure is used, it's important that the open portion of the wound not be electrocoagulated or treated with chemical styptics. Bleeding should be controlled with pressure and/or packing with absorbable material. Sutures can usually be removed in three to five days.

Wound closure with dissolving sutures

Removing sutures from a skin wound inconveniences the patient and is a time-consuming nuisance for the physician. Why not use dissolving sutures for skin closure? Synthetic absorbable sutures have drawbacks when used on the skin, but gut works surprisingly well. Webster and his plastic surgical colleagues reported that "for many years we have used 6-0 catgut for closure of epithelial and superficial dermal wound edges."[4] They emphasize that not all gut sutures are suitable, preferring 6-0 Davis and Geck mild chromic gut, but also finding 6-0 plain gut sutures from Ethicon suitable. (My experience has been limited to the products of these two companies.) I'm not aware of other published studies, although I know a number of dermatologic surgeons routinely use gut for skin closure.

Cosmetic results are comparable to traditional suture technique, provided that fine sutures and tape support are used (Figures C-1 through C-4). Complications (wound infection or dehiscence) are as rare as with traditional techniques. Drawbacks? Gut suture is stiff, so suturing takes a little longer. There is significant variation in dissolution (breakage) time from patient to patient; allow for this. Used alone, gut sutures are not reliable for closing wounds under heavy tension.

Gut sutures provide wound support only while intact. Following breakage, gut suture remnants remain in the skin until shed as a result of removal of the tape support, washing, or ordinary wear and tear. The remnants cause remarkably little skin reaction.

Breakage (dissolving) time varies with suture, patient, and the degree of wound tension. The coarser the suture, the longer it remains intact. Sutures will usually break within the following times:

6-0 plain gut (Ethicon)	3 to 7 days
6-0 mild chromic gut (Davis and Geck)	5 to 12 days
5-0 plain gut (Ethicon)	5 to 12 days
4-0 plain gut (Ethicon)	9 to 20 days

Practical points

I use gut suture supported with "paper" tape applied over spirit gum adhecasive. Following wound closure and cessation of bleeding, spirit gum adhesive is painted on the wound edges up to the suture line. Nonsterile, flesh-colored "paper" tape is applied to "tent up" the wound edges slightly and take tension off the wound (Figure C-3). The dressing is completed with gauze to cover the "paper" tape. The gauze bandage is removed the next day, and the tape is allowed to remain in place for two to three weeks. The suture remnants usually come off when the tape separates. Follow-up care is detailed in the patient information sheet titled "Care of Wounds Closed With Dissolving Stitches."

In hairy areas, prolonged tape support is not feasible. No dressing is used on the scalp after cyst removal. On the beard area, the patient is told to remove the tape gently when it is loosened by the beard growth and leave the wound open thereafter.

On the face I generally use 6-0 mild chromic gut. If there is an area of no tension—such as the eyelids—I use 6-0 plain gut. If there is moderate tension on the face, a combination of mattress sutures of 5-0 plain gut and interrupted sutures of 6-0 mild chromic gut is useful. On the scalp and trunk I use either 5-0 or 4-0 plain gut. When there is significant wound tension, it must be relieved with buried subcuticular sutures of polyglycolic acid or polyglactin prior to gut closure.

It is important to use either plain gut or 6-0 *mild* chromic gut of Davis and Geck. Regular chromic gut is absorbed far too slowly from the skin. I've

Dermatologic surgery

found that even Davis and Geck 5-0 mild chromic gut may remain in the skin inordinately long.

Patients like this approach to skin closure because it spares them the nuisance and waste of time of a second office visit—a major benefit for out-of-town patients. For patients going on a trip, it saves the need to search out a physician for suture removal. It eliminates the frequent, though groundless, fear of stitch removal.

You will like gut suture skin closure because it's a significant timesaver, especially if just a few sutures are placed for cyst removal (Figure C-15), biopsy, or a small excision. You can perform surgery a few days before going on vacation, and check on the nicely healed wound after you return! Give it a try on a few small wounds at first. I predict it will convert you to using it on larger ones.

Electrocoagulation of small blood vessels

Vascular spiders and other small dermal blood vessels are best treated by electrocoagulation using a bipolar current. The bipolar current is definitely superior to a monopolar current in treating these lesions. A small, pointed needle that can penetrate skin is required. Either a commercial epilating needle or a 27- to 30-gauge hypodermic needle is suitable.

Adjust the apparatus for bipolar coagulation at a low to medium setting to produce a spark about 1 to 2 mm between needle and ground electrode. The patient then firmly grasps the ground electrode between his hands. With the current *off,* plunge the point of the needle several millimeters into the skin, to the estimated depth of the vascular lesion. Then turn the current on briefly. The vessel should blanch. If it doesn't, increase the current's intensity and repeat the treatment. Treat remaining vascular branches in the same manner. Under no condition should there be any surface sparking or surface necrosis. Should surface sparking occur, it means you're using too strong a current or the patient isn't adequately grounded.

The aim of this treatment is to produce a small, deep scar that destroys the blood vessel but is invisibly small. The bipolar current enables deep destruction with sparing of the epidermis. More than one treatment is often necessary. Sometimes it's impossible to eradicate a vascular spider in this manner. Until the physician becomes experienced with this technique, he should be very cautious and err on the side of too low a current. You can always repeat the treatment.

References

1. Stegman SJ, Tromovitch TA, Glogau RG: *Basics of Dermatologic Surgery.* Chicago: Year Book Medical Publishers, 1982

2. Epstein, Ervin, and Epstein, Ervin Jr: *Techniques in Skin Surgery.* Philadelphia: Lea & Febiger, 1979

3. Epstein E: Surgery of skin tumors: Excision with partial suture closure. *Cutis* 18:384, 1976

4. Webster RC, Davidson TM, Smith RC: Wound closure with absorbable sutures. *Laryngoscope* 86:1280, 1976

4

Acne

Etiology

Acne, an inflammatory disorder of the sebaceous glands, is exceedingly common among teen-agers and frequently continues into adulthood. The fact that innumerable remedies are advertised to the medical profession and to patients indicates that none is satisfactory.

Certain drugs, notably the iodides and bromides, but also systemic corticosteroids, can produce acneiform eruptions. Acneiform eruptions may be caused or aggravated by externally applied fluorinated hydrocarbons, cutting oils, pomades, and other greasy materials.

Diagnosis

The appearance of acne is distinctive, and diagnosis is usually easy. Rosacea (acne rosacea) has some resemblance to acne but lacks comedones, has patchy erythema, and preferentially affects the middle-aged and elderly. The poorly understood syndrome known as perioral dermatitis has acneiform papules and pustules but, unlike adult acne, also has patches of low-grade dermatitis. Isolated deep inflammatory lesions—acne abscesses—may be indistinguishable from furuncles or inflamed cysts.

Treatment

Most textbooks make acne therapy sound simple and logical. It is neither. There are myriad treatments, each with champions and detractors. Although many dermatologists proclaim their success in treating acne, our patients are less convinced. It's common to encounter patients distressed because their continuing acne hasn't benefited from consultation with several dermatologists.

Noninflammatory acne lesions

The therapy of noninflammatory lesions differs from that of inflammatory lesions. Comedones (blackheads) and closed comedones (whiteheads) are noninflammatory lesions. They usually cause little distress. These lesions can be removed mechanically with comedo extractors and a fine needle or pointed blade to open closed comedones. Such maneuvers are temporary; new comedones form promptly. Many dermatologists believe—without proof—that mechanically removing comedones prevents the formation of inflammatory lesions. My belief is that mechanical removal is worthless.

I play down the significance of comedones to see whether patients are willing to ignore them. Most patients are content to live with their blackheads once they understand they are not caused by dirt and do not exacerbate their acne. I encourage women to hide them with water-based makeup.

Some patients do request treatment. Certain peeling and irritating agents will decrease the number of comedones. The most effective is retinoic acid (Retin-A). It's irritating and should be used cautiously. Patients are directed to apply the 0.025 per cent gel or 0.05 per cent cream sparingly at bedtime to areas of blackheads until irritation occurs, and then to use it every second or third night. Some patients are satisfied; others find it difficult to eradicate blackheads without excessive irritation. As with any other acne treatment, its benefit is temporary.

Inflammatory lesions

The inflammatory lesions of acne—papules and pustules—are what really concern the patient. The many therapies currently in vogue, and my assessment of their effectiveness, are summarized in Table 4-1. All current acne therapies are of temporary benefit only. Since acne medications only suppress acne, they should be continued for months or years until acne undergoes spontaneous resolution.

The therapeutic measures outlined in Table 4-1 differ; some aim to hasten involution of established lesions, while the intent of others is to prevent new lesions. Thus intralesional corticosteroids, while subduing the lesions injected, don't prevent the development of fresh lesions. Effective systemic antibiotic therapy does suppress the formation of new inflammatory lesions—a result patients prefer.

At present, only systemic antibiotics, isotretinoin (13-*cis*-retinoic acid), and topical antimicrobials have been shown to be effective in suppressing acne. Of these three, systemic antibiotics are by far the most useful. Isotretinoin, a vitamin A derivative, is often effective against severe nodulocystic acne that has failed to respond to systemic antibiotics. It has the additional advantage of prolonged improvement after therapy ends. But because of its significant toxicity, it won't replace systemic antibiotics as the mainstay of acne therapy. Isotretinoin is a potent teratogen, frequently causes increases in serum lipids, and almost always produces cutaneous side effects, including cheilitis, nosebleeds, stomatitis, and xerosis.

Topical therapy
Topical antibiotics for acne are an exciting new approach since they combine proven effectiveness with cosmetic elegance. The currently available prep-

TABLE 4-1

Summary of treatment of inflammatory acne

Topical therapy	Effectiveness
Topical antibiotics—special formulations	+
Benzoyl peroxide	+
Sulfur, resorcinol, and salicylic acid	?
Retinoic acid	0
Medicated soaps and cleansers	0
Abradant cleansers	0
Acetone, alcohol, and other "degreasing" lotions	0
Systemic therapy	
Antibiotics	+
13-*cis*-Retinoic acid (isotretinoin)	+
Corticosteroids	(+)sp
Sex hormones	(+)sp
Vitamins	0
Office procedures	
Acne surgery	(+)sp
Intralesional corticosteroids	+
Cryotherapy	?
Ultraviolet therapy	0
X-ray therapy	*
Miscellaneous	
Psychological factors	+
Sunshine	†
Diet	?
Skin hygiene	0
Nervous tension	?
Cosmetics	?

KEY:
+ = effective
(+)sp = effective in certain special situations
? = possibly slightly effective
0 = no benefit

*X-ray therapy has been proven effective in suppressing acne.
In my opinion, its risks outweigh its benefits.
†Many but not all acne patients benefit from sunlight.

arations are tetracycline (Topicycline), erythromycin (A/T/S lotion, Ery-Derm lotion, Staticin), clindamycin (Cleocin T lotion), and meclocycline sulfosalicylate (Meclan cream). Topical clindamycin has caused rare cases of diarrhea and colitis; the others are free of systemic side effects.

Which topical antibiotic should you prescribe? It's difficult to offer firm guidelines because the field is continually changing. Since adequate comparison trials are lacking, I use the topical antibiotics my patients like. Topical tetracycline leaves a colored residue on the skin, and its vehicle sometimes is irritating. I avoid it. All the topical erythromycins and topical

Acne

clindamycin have hydroalcoholic vehicles, which most patients tolerate well. Staticin contains a substance that's irritating to some patients. For patients with dry or irritable skin, I favor the use of topical meclocycline because of its cream vehicle.

Of the nonantibiotic antimicrobials, benzoyl peroxide deserves mention because many dermatologists swear by it. It's a potent antimicrobial available in a wide variety of creams, gels, and liquids. It tends to irritate and occasionally causes contact allergy. Since the topical antibiotics are superior, I don't use benzoyl peroxide.

Sulfur, resorcinol, and salicylic acid are the classical time-tested topical agents. The fact that none of these has ever been shown effective in controlled studies hasn't prevented their extensive use in both over-the-counter and prescription acne remedies.

Topicals containing retinoic acid, while of proven effectiveness in treating comedones and other noninflammatory lesions, have been disappointing in the therapy of inflammatory acne.

There is no evidence that special soaps, abradant cleansers, astringents, and similar products are of benefit in inflammatory acne. I tell patients they are a waste of money and advise ordinary soap and water for cleansing. Overenthusiastic use of acne cleansers may lead to a low-grade facial irritant dermatitis.

Systemic therapy

Antibiotics. At present, systemic antibiotics are the most common therapy for acne. The practical aspects deserve a detailed discussion.

Start with tetracycline. Keep in mind that there is no "standard" dosage of tetracycline in acne, and that not all persons respond to tetracycline. A few do well on as little as 250 to 500 mg of tetracycline a day; however, the majority will require 1 gm or more to show a satisfactory result. The response of acne to antibiotics is gradual, and it takes six weeks to determine whether the medication is of benefit.

For new patients not previously treated with systemic antibiotics, initiate therapy with a six-week course of 1 gm of tetracycline a day. The drug is taken in two 500-mg doses with water on an empty stomach, once on arising and once in the evening; tell the patient to avoid dairy products within an hour of ingesting tetracycline. Mention the possibility of yeast vaginitis to women, and advise them to call your office if they develop genital itching and a vaginal discharge. At the six-week follow-up visit, the patient's skin will be (1) greatly improved, (2) partially, but definitely, better, (3) unchanged or equivocal, or (4) worse.

The dramatically improved patient is a delight, but in the minority. Improvement usually continues for another six to eight weeks on the same dosage. After that, gradual reduction may be attempted. To find the smallest effective daily dose of tetracycline, have the patient decrease his daily ration by 250 mg at four- to six-week intervals. When the acne flares up, he should return to the dose that previously controlled it. This attempt to reduce the dose should be repeated. I generally prescribe a four-month supply of tetracycline and ask the patient to return before it's used up. The patient instruction sheet explains the details of this gradual decrease and lets you write in a suggested schedule.

When there's a partial response, I generally increase the tetracycline to 1.5 gm a day, usually as 750 mg taken twice daily. Patients should be warned about the phototoxic effect of tetracycline, which is dose-related. In sunny climes, 1.5 gm of tetracycline a day will cause easy sunburning in many individuals. The patient returns in six weeks for another evaluation. When the partial response to tetracycline is fairly satisfactory, I frequently have the patient continue on the same dose (1 gm a day) for two to three months. If there is some response to tetracycline in six weeks, the same dose will usually produce additional benefit over the succeeding months.

When there is an equivocal response or failure, you have the arbitrary choice of trying a higher dose of tetracycline or changing to another antibiotic. Except during the summer months, I tend to use a higher dose of tetracycline. During the summer, or if the patient asks for another antibiotic, I use erythromycin.

When the patient's acne is worse after a trial of tetracycline, it should be explained that this was not the result of the tetracycline, but that the acne was in a spontaneously worsening phase. Antibiotics do not aggravate acne, except for the rare complication of gram-negative folliculitis.

The commonest complication of tetracycline therapy is yeast vaginitis. There are no hard data as to its frequency, but I estimate it occurs in about 10 per cent of female acne patients receiving 1 gm of tetracycline daily. Women should be routinely warned about it. The appearance of genital itching and a vaginal discharge is an indication for specific anticandidal therapy; however, the tetracycline should be continued. My method of managing this complication is to prescribe an anticandidal preparation—nystatin (Mycostatin, Nilstat), candicidin (Vanobid), or clotrimazole (Gyne-Lotrimin, Mycelex-G)—with the instructions that if the symptoms don't clear rapidly she is to consult her general physician or gynecologist for the proper pelvic examination. Not all cases of vaginitis are caused by yeast.

Phototoxicity is the second most common complication. Patients taking 250 to 500 mg daily rarely experience it. On 1 gm a day, in sunny climates, many patients will sunburn easily. At 2 gm daily almost all patients will burn easily and must be warned to take appropriate sun-protective measures. I routinely hand them a sheet describing sun protection. The hands are frequently the site of sunburn, and photo-onycholysis—separation of the nail plate from its bed as a result of sunshine—is an occasional, distressing occurrence. Fortunately, it's reversible.

Gastrointestinal distress occurs occasionally. Usually it's temporary. Try having the patient divide his daily tetracycline ration into four doses rather than two. If there are still problems, start with one tetracycline capsule a day and see if this dose can gradually be increased. If the gastrointestinal distress persists, or if there is severe presternal burning or discomfort (heartburn), stop the tetracycline. Esophageal erosions may have occurred. Tetracycline taken at bedtime seems to be the common denominator in this complication. It's a good idea to advise patients to take their tetracycline *before* bedtime and with a full glass of water.

Blistering of the sun-exposed extremities and face, producing a porphyria-like clinical picture, is a rare complication. If this occurs, stop the tetracycline. Colitis as a complication of tetracycline therapy in otherwise healthy acne patients is exceedingly rare. However, if a patient complains that tetracycline gives him diarrhea, stop the drug.

Tetracycline should be discontinued if the patient becomes pregnant, as the drug is incorporated into the fetal bones and teeth. Tetracycline is contraindicated in children under 8 years because it discolors the permanent teeth—but acne is rare in this age group. In patients with inadequate renal function, tetraycycline should not be used. Some physicians periodically perform blood counts and urinalyses on patients taking long-term tetracycline. There doesn't seem to be any rationale for this.

Alternative antibiotics. What if tetracycline fails—even when given in doses as high as 2 to 3 gm a day? Try another antibiotic. There's no rational way of choosing an alternative antibiotic; everyone has his favorites. I use erythromycin if tetracycline fails or produces annoying side effects. Erythromycin has been used for many years, is remarkably safe, and does not cause photosensitivity. Like other antibiotics, it may cause yeast vaginitis. Erythromycin appears to cause more gastrointestinal intolerance than tetracycline. However, there are several forms of erythromycin that can be taken with food, and this reduces the incidence of gastrointestinal side effects. One salt of erythromycin, the estolate, may cause hepatic dysfunction and should not be used in the treatment of acne.

If neither tetracycline nor erythromycin is effective, I prescribe minocycline. Start with 100 mg a day; if there is no response, cautiously increase this to 150 or possibly 200 mg a day. The chief adverse effect of minocycline is dizziness. It's dose-related, and rare on a daily dose of 100 mg or less. Very rarely, prolonged use of minocycline colors the skin gray or blue-black; this effect is reversible. Minocycline is well tolerated by the gastrointestinal tract and may be taken with meals. It's not a significant photosensitizer, but is expensive.

If adequate doses of tetracycline, erythromycin, and minocycline all fail—and this is not uncommon—my next step is trimethoprim-sulfamethoxazole (Bactrim, Septra). The usual dose is one regular-strength tablet twice daily. When the patient improves, the dose is gradually reduced. This combination is sometimes effective when many other antimicrobials have failed. Remember that it contains a sulfonamide, and sulfonamides are riskier drugs than antibiotics. Blood dyscrasias are the most serious potential adverse reactions, so periodic blood counts are essential. Sulfonamides occasionally produce severe allergic reactions. Before starting therapy, ask the patient about previous experience with sulfa drugs.

Clindamycin is effective against acne; unfortunately, it occasionally causes severe pseudomembranous colitis. Most dermatologists reserve clindamycin for severe, "life-ruining" acne not helped by other antibiotics.

Corticosteroids. Properly used, systemic corticosteroids may be of great benefit in severe acne. There is a rare, severe, febrile acne, usually accompanied by arthralgia, that responds poorly to antibiotics and often improves with systemic corticosteroids. Corticosteroids in acne must be used properly, since continual moderate to high doses of systemic corticosteroids may actually cause acne (steroid acne). Corticosteroids should be used for as brief a time as possible, a short-acting form such as prednisone employed, and the patient weaned to an every-other-day or every-third-day regimen. Occasionally, moderate to severe acne that responds poorly to antibiotics will benefit greatly from a month or two of prednisone taken as a single morning dose of 20 mg two or three times a week. This regimen seems safe and will sometimes tide a patient over a bout of severe acne.

Topical corticosteroids are without value in acne. Fluorinated corticosteroids may aggravate acne and should not be used on the face of a patient with acne. If seborrheic dermatitis coexists with acne—a fairly common combination—prescribe 1 per cent hydrocortisone lotion or cream.

Sex hormones. Estrogens and estrogen-dominant birth-control pills are often beneficial against acne in women. It isn't uncommon for acne to appear in adult women who have stopped taking an estrogen-dominant contraceptive. Whether cessation of the pill triggered acne, or whether the hormone had been suppressing adult acne present all along, is not known. Androgen-dominant birth-control pills may aggravate acne. In many women oral contraceptives have no effect on acne. Estrogen therapy and birth-control pills have significant medical side effects. The risk-benefit ratio rarely justifies the use of oral contraceptives for treating acne.

Vitamins. Vitamin A by mouth has had a long and undeserved vogue in acne therapy. It is without value. As high doses may be toxic, it should not be used. Vitamins are worthless in acne.

Zinc. In pharmacologic doses, zinc can suppress acne. Its effect is relatively weak, roughly equivalent to low doses of systemic antibiotics. We know nothing about zinc's long-term toxicity. Over the short term there may be gastrointestinal irritation and ulcers. Although zinc is touted as a "natural" treatment for acne, I shun it. Systemic antibiotics are more effective, and we know they're safe for long-term use.

Office procedures

Acne surgery

Acne surgery refers to several manipulative approaches, including removal of comedones, needling acne lesions, and incising acne lesions or abscesses with a small pointed blade. Incising fluctuant lesions for drainage used to be popular; with the advent of intralesional corticosteroids, this method is used less often. Incising a lesion may leave a small scar; injecting a corticosteroid does not. I incise only the rare large, fluctuant acne lesions that don't respond to intralesional corticosteroids. When a large acne abscess requires drainage, after local anesthesia make a 2- to 3-mm-long incision with a pointed No. 11 blade and gently scoop out the necrotic material with a 1-mm-diameter chalazion curette. The incision should be made parallel to the wrinkle lines of the face; if the procedure is cautiously performed, scarring is infrequent.

Many dermatologists like to express comedones and open closed comedones regularly. When these procedures are done gently, they don't leave scars. However, there's no evidence that they prevent inflammatory lesions. Many patients who have had such acne surgery elsewhere seem relieved if told they won't be "picked on."

Intralesional corticosteroids

These work. Injecting a diluted suspension of repository corticosteroid into a papulopustule leads to improvement within a day or two, with flattening of the lesion (Figures C-5 and C-6). Flat lesions are more readily camouflaged with makeup or a tinted acne lotion. When a 30-gauge needle is used, there's little discomfort. Triamcinolone acetonide suspension is the agent generally employed; use it in a dilution to 2 to 3 mg/ml. Higher concentrations may cause temporary skin atrophy and an annoying depression at the site of injection. Inject 0.02 to 0.04 ml at a depth of 4 to 5 mm (about one-third the length of a half-inch-long needle) as described in Chapter 1.

In the United States, the most dilute suspension of triamcinolone acetonide commercially available is 10 mg/ml. You will need to make (or have the pharmacy do it) a diluted triamcinolone acetonide suspension. This can be prepared by using 30-ml vials of preservative-containing saline (labeled "multiple dose" saline); after removing and discarding 10 ml of saline, add 5 ml of triamcinolone acetonide suspension 10 mg/ml. Intralesional therapy is useful as the sole method of treatment of intermittent acne. It's helpful as an adjunct when acne is not adequately suppressed with antibiotics.

Cryotherapy

Cryotherapy with Dry Ice or liquid nitrogen has been used for years for its peeling and desquamating effect. It reduces the number of comedones and closed comedones and may hasten the involution of existing papulopustules. Cryotherapy does not prevent new inflammatory lesions. Its action is dramatic: It stings considerably at the time of application, and redness persists 6 to 12 hours after treatment. I have found the benefits less dramatic and abandoned it. However, many competent dermatologists consider cryotherapy an effective modality.

Ultraviolet light therapy

Ultraviolet sunlamps have enjoyed popularity because of the observation that sunlight benefits many acne patients. Sunlamps, however, don't produce light of the same wavelengths emitted by the sun and so they fail to duplicate sunlight's beneficial effect. This doesn't prevent many patients and physicians from using ultraviolet lamps; there's no doubt that the tanning—and occasional burns—can be a potent placebo.

X-ray therapy

Briefly mentioned, only to be dismissed, is X-ray therapy. Although superficial X-ray therapy will temporarily suppress acne vulgaris, such therapy may damage skin and in some persons lead eventually to an increased tendency to form skin cancers. There is widespread skepticism as to whether X-ray therapy is justified for a benign process. To me, X-ray therapy for acne is of only historical interest.

Managing the patient

Psychological factors

Skillful psychological management rivals only systemic antibiotics in its importance as a treatment modality. It's hard for an adult to realize how distressing even trivial acne may be to teen-agers. The physician must show (or at least try to show) sympathetic interest in the patient's problem and not deal with an acne patient as a nuisance to be gotten rid of as soon as possible. Granted, this is often difficult.

Find out the patient's expectations. A wise dermatologist used to ask new acne patients, "Do you expect me to cure your acne?" When they answered yes, he gently told them there was no cure for acne, but "I will help you." Be honest and admit the present unsatisfactory state of acne treatment; the patient will find out soon enough.

Tell patients that treatment suppresses acne but does not cure it. Only nature and time will do this. Don't provide a timetable for patients to outgrow their acne; we see too many adults reassured by a previous physician that their "teen-age" acne would stop at an age they passed long ago.

Help the patient put his acne into perspective. Point out that when he looks at himself in a mirror, he sees only his unsightly pimples; when others view him, they see the entire person, and it's the looks of the whole "package" that count. Mention some physically attractive aspect—a woman's pretty hair or figure, a man's rugged physique. This support is all the psychotherapy most acne patients need.

Intralesional repository corticosteroid therapy is a useful "crutch" for acne sufferers. Tell them that rather than worry about a disfiguring crop of pimples just before an important job interview, date, or other stressful occasion, they can have them injected for prompt relief. Knowing about the availability of this emergency approach enables many patients to tolerate their acne better.

Many patients—and their parents—believe that acne is a result of some incorrect habit or cleansing method. You can lift this burden of guilt from patients' shoulders by pointing out that there's little patients can do, without a prescription, either to benefit or to aggravate their acne. I tell them that sunlight is the only effective nonprescription acne treatment. Patients are reassured that, except for picking, there is little that worsens acne. The other exception is eating a food that they find triggers acne flare-ups.

Picking deserves special attention in patients with crusted, excoriated, or otherwise manipulated lesions (Figure C-7). This is more common in young women, and seems to be an outgrowth of misguided attempts to "scrub away" their pimples. Patients should be told emphatically not to pick, squeeze, or otherwise manipulate their pimples. When a crop of pimples renders a patient desperate, I advise him or her to hide them with some flesh-colored, water-based makeup or use a flesh-tinted acne lotion.

Treating acne is often discouraging for the physician as well as the patient. Many patients derive great benefit from the support of a sympathetic and concerned physician in spite of little objective improvement in their acne. Remember, time is usually on your side.

Sunshine

Sunshine benefits most acne patients. Some cases fail to improve with sunlight, and a small minority are even aggravated. Unfortunately, sunlight also causes gradual, irreversible skin damage; consequently, most dermatologists have mixed feelings about recommending sunbaths for acne. Short-term acne benefits have to be weighed against the long-term risks of skin aging and skin cancer.

Diet

One can find all shades of opinion on the relationship of diet to acne, little of it supported by documented observations. Although chocolate has a notorious reputation for aggravating acne, attempts to show such effects have failed. A reasonable approach is to tell patients that foods do not cause acne, but that in some cases certain foods may aggravate it. Chocolate, nuts, cola drinks, and root beer are the aggravators of acne most commonly cited by patients. I alert patients to these potential aggravators and suggest that they observe whether repeated flare-ups occur after they consume these foods. If so, they are asked to stop them. Occasionally, large quantities of milk aggravate acne—usually this means 2 to 3 liters a day. Patients consuming such large quantities of milk are asked to stop their milk intake for three to four weeks and then resume it again as a test to determine its role.

Skin hygiene

Most acne patients have been indoctrinated in the importance of skin hygiene for care of their complexions. Many engage in lengthy, expensive, and sometimes irritating cleansing and scrubbing routines. This is worthless, and patients should be told that while cleanliness may be next to godliness, it doesn't help acne. Advise patients to wash with ordinary soap and water once or twice a day and forget about abradants, astringents, medicated soaps, degreasing pads, and so on. Point out that it is not the surface oil that causes acne, but the oil that doesn't get to the surface. Stress that acne is not caused by dirt.

Nervous tension

It's easy to blame "nerves" for acne and thus subtly shift the blame for therapeutic failure from the physician to the patient. Emotional upsets and nervous tension may aggravate acne, just as emotional factors can worsen hypertension, diabetes, rheumatoid arthritis, and a host of other organic disorders. Reassure the patient that emotional stresses and worry sometimes aggravate acne but never cause it. Patients often feel guilty and responsible for their acne. We should relieve feelings of guilt, not add to them. Emotional stresses cause patients to become more aware of their acne and sometimes to excoriate or otherwise aggravate it physically. Explain this to patients and tell them gently but firmly not to pick, squeeze, scratch, or otherwise manipulate their pimples.

Cosmetics

Thick, greasy cosmetics such as actors' makeup can aggravate acne. Beyond that, little is certain. Some dermatologists consider cosmetics a major cause of the all-too-common acne of adult women; others believe their effect is insignificant. From observing women with adult acne who abstained from all cosmetics for many months, I've concluded that cosmetics usually play little role in papulopustular (inflammatory) lesions. Consequently I permit acne patients the use of makeup, provided they use water-based cosmetics and thoroughly wash them off at night with soap and water, not a cold cream. However, I warn them that cosmetics and sunscreens can sometimes cause acne flare-ups.

Summary

The status of acne therapy is still unsatisfactory. Acne patients are full of concerns, questions, and misconceptions. Educating and counseling patients takes time; a patient instruction form is invaluable in managing acne. The instruction form accompanying this unit is tailored to my understanding of what represents effective acne therapy; you may wish to modify it. Treating acne is vexing but, when successful, enormously gratifying.

Patient sheets pages P-7, P-35, P-59, P-61, P-63, P-65, P-67, P-79

Actinic keratoses

5

Etiology

Actinic keratoses are the visible consequences of sunlight (actinic) damage to skin cells. They're restricted to the sun-exposed portions of the skin and are particularly common in the fair-skinned populations of sunny climes. I have never seen them in a dark-skinned black.

Diagnosis

Diagnosis is usually straightforward—the scaly, often red, irregularly surfaced, sharply demarcated roughenings on the sun-exposed areas of fair-skinned persons are distinctive.

The main differential diagnostic considerations are warts, seborrheic keratoses, Bowen's disease (intraepidermal squamous-cell carcinoma), and basal- or squamous-cell carcinoma. Excluding malignancy is the most troublesome problem. When the lesion is infiltrated or moderately deep, precise clinical diagnosis is impossible and tissue examination is needed. Some diagnostic uncertainty vis-à-vis carcinoma always exists, even in superficial lesions. For this reason, any keratosis that recurs after treatment should be biopsied.

Coexisting dermatitis such as psoriasis or seborrheic dermatitis may be impossible to distinguish clinically from superficial actinic keratoses. In this situation I treat the dermatitis vigorously with a topical corticosteroid for two to three weeks and then re-evaluate the patient's condition. The dermatitis usually responds to this regimen, while actinic keratoses undergo relatively little change.

Treatment

Patients usually seek treatment because they find the lesions unsightly or are concerned about potential malignancy. Most actinic keratoses are superficial; superficial destruction of the defective skin cells is all that's needed.

There are three treatments of choice: (1) superficial surgical removal with curette and/or scissors, (2) liquid nitrogen freezing, and (3) topical 5-fluorouracil (5-FU). Treatment must be individualized.

Cosmetic results are best with topical 5-FU because it selectively destroys actinically damaged cells. The second-best cosmetic results are achieved by superficial liquid nitrogen freezing. Cosmetic results after curettage are usually inferior to the other two methods, but if the curettage is carefully done the scar is often invisible. Note that I didn't mention electrodesiccation as a treatment. Although widely used, it frequently leaves unsightly scars.

Superficial surgical removal of actinic keratoses is readily accomplished by curettage as described in Chapter 3. Sometimes protuberant lesions, especially on the hands, are best snipped off with scissors. Depending on cosmetic considerations and the depth of the lesion, bleeding is controlled with or without styptics and the patient given the appropriate instruction form. Caution patients who have had keratoses removed from the lower leg that healing will be prolonged.

The great advantage of superficial surgical removal is that it provides tissue for possible histologic examination. Note that "possible." When numerous keratoses are removed by curettage, it's unreasonable to submit all of them for histology. It suffices to submit the deep lesions. Sometimes the curette "falls" deeply into a lesion presumed to be superficial. This suggests malignancy; have the tissue examined by a pathologist.

Liquid nitrogen is particularly useful in patients who return repeatedly with crops of multiple actinic keratoses. If you don't use liquid nitrogen, I suggest you refer these patients to someone who does. The technique of liquid nitrogen treatment is described in Chapter 3; you should give the patient the postoperative instruction sheet for liquid nitrogen treatment. The main drawback of liquid nitrogen treatment is that one relies entirely on a clinical diagnosis. Since actinic keratoses are sometimes indistinguishable from carcinoma, adequate follow-up is mandatory. If a keratosis doesn't clear up with liquid nitrogen treatment, biopsy it. This is best accomplished by superficial scissors or curette removal, which also cures benign lesions. With this limitation in mind, liquid nitrogen remains the best treatment for patients who continue to develop multiple actinic keratoses.

Topical 5-FU is the method of choice when there are myriads of actinic keratoses. It's an effective way of removing one or a few keratoses when they are superficial and the optimum cosmetic result is desired. As with liquid nitrogen, the treatment is based on clinical diagnosis without histologic control. Whereas liquid nitrogen destroys such superficial neoplasms as seborrheic keratoses and warts, topical 5-FU does not.

Topical formulations of 5-FU are available in the United States from Herbert Laboratories and Roche Laboratories. One firm produces a 1 per cent solution and a 1 per cent cream; the other, 2 per cent and 5 per cent solutions and a 5 per cent cream. The choice of formulation isn't critical. The solutions seem to work somewhat more rapidly—and also irritate normal skin more—than the creams. Whichever formulation is used, the patient applies it until the physician has judged that enough destruction has occurred—usually

Actinic keratoses

when the lesions have ulcerated. Then the skin is allowed to heal. Often a lubricant aids patient comfort during this process.

Topical 5-FU produces raw, inflamed areas that are unsightly and often uncomfortable. This stage lasts two to four weeks and often leads to bitter complaints. When informing patients about 5-FU therapy, be sure to show them photographs (available from the manufacturers) of what happens during treatments.

Topical 5-FU, while effective in destroying actinic keratoses of the face, usually fails to remove keratoses of the hands and forearms. Combining topical retinoic acid (Retin-A and other brands) with topical 5-FU produces a potentiating effect sufficient to destroy actinic keratoses of the hands and forearms. This combined treatment also works on the legs; however, keratoses of the legs seem to take forever to heal, and I usually avoid using the combined 5-FU-retinoic acid treatment there.

Step-by-step directions for using 5-FU follow. While this is the technique I use, other schedules are equally effective.

1. Topical 5-FU is applied three times a day with the finger to the actinic keratotic areas of the face and massaged in well. Most brochures suggest twice-a-day usage, but applying it three times a day speeds things up.
2. The medicine is to be applied to the entire sun-damaged area—the entire forehead, cheek, or face—not just to individual keratoses. The reason for this is that topical 5-FU will destroy early keratoses not clinically evident.
3. When applying 5-FU the patient should avoid (1) the eyelids, (2) the folds about the nose, and (3) the lips, as 5-FU is irritating in these locations. Exceptions are made when specific lesions in these regions need to be destroyed.
4. Have patients avoid the sun during treatment. Give them specific written instructions on the patient information sheet and inform them that in three to five days the treated areas will become red.
5. The patient returns in 7 to 10 days.
6. At the one-week follow-up visit, most patients have developed early erosions and should continue the medication for another 10 to 14 days, depending on how severe the reaction is. For patients using the 5 per cent solution three times daily, 14 to 21 days of treatment usually suffice. The cream formulations usually require a week longer. Certain areas—notably the forehead and scalp—may need longer treatment than more sensitive areas such as the lower cheeks and mouth. If at one week there's little response, the patient continues the treatment and returns a week later.
7. The patient is given a definite stopping date for the treatment, which is written out for him. After 5-FU has been stopped, white petrolatum may be applied thinly at bedtime to soothe raw areas while they heal. The patient returns after six weeks for final evaluation.
8. In treating actinic keratoses of the hands and forearms, the patient applies 0.1 per cent retinoic acid solution in the morning to the entire sun-damaged area with a cotton-tipped applicator. In the afternoon and at bedtime 5 per cent 5-FU cream is applied and thoroughly massaged in. To avoid confusion, it's simplest to use the retinoic acid as a solution and the 5-FU as a

cream. The patient returns at weekly intervals. When marked erosions appear, the retinoic acid is stopped and only 5-FU cream is continued three times daily for an additional 7 to 14 days. The entire 5-FU treatment takes significantly longer on the hands and forearms than on the face.

9. Some patients prefer to treat one area of the face at a time to minimize the extent of the cosmetic handicap. With an intelligent patient this usually works. I follow such patients through one area until it's completely healed, and then instruct them to proceed the same way systematically to other areas, pushing the treatment to rawness and then stopping. Emphasize that they are not to treat any area twice and that you should evaluate any lesions that fail to respond to a single course of 5-FU. Ask these patients to return after they have completed their entire spot-by-spot treatment.

10. At the final follow-up visit, residual lesions should be destroyed. If you're confident that they're benign—for instance, seborrheic keratoses are not removed by topical 5-FU—liquid nitrogen is fine. However, suspect any actinic keratosis that fails to respond to adequate 5-FU treatment as being a carcinoma; it's best treated by curette removal and the tissue should be analyzed histologically. It's a mistake to use a second course of 5-FU on lesions that failed to respond the first time. On the other hand, it's both permissible and useful to re-treat patients with topical 5-FU a year or more later if new keratoses appear.

Actinic keratoses

6

Alopecia areata

Etiology

Alopecia areata is a fairly common skin disorder. While a frequent familial pattern indicates that genetic factors play a role, the cause of alopecia areata remains unknown. The slightly increased incidence of thyroid disorders and vitiligo in alopecia areata points in the direction of autosensitization. While textbooks and lay publications frequently stress the role of emotional factors, this is not a psychogenic disorder. Patients shouldn't be made to feel responsible for their "nerves" causing the alopecia.

Diagnosis

Diagnosis of typical cases is easy; the round, sharply demarcated patches of complete hair loss are characteristic. Keep in mind that alopecia areata is characterized by a defect in hair growth. Structurally defective hairs are usually visible on close inspection. Diagnostic is the "exclamation-point hair," a short hair that's thinner at its base than at the top and represents the last gasp of a hair follicle prior to inactivity. If hair at the edges of the patch pulls out easily and has clubbed ends, it helps confirm the diagnosis and indicates that the process is active and the patch will enlarge.

The two chief differential diagnoses are tinea capitis and trichotillomania. In tinea capitis, scaling and inflammation of the scalp are often evident. Examination under Wood's (black) light and microscopy of KOH-cleared broken-off hairs are useful in excluding tinea capitis. Unfortunately, both techniques are often misinterpreted; one must be careful not to interpret Wood's light fluorescence of debris, or the normal mild scalp fluorescence, as tinea. Trichotillomania usually shows broken-off, normal-appearing, growing-stage hair. At times it's difficult to distinguish alopecia areata from trichotillomania except by observation over time.

Alopecia areata sometimes fails to produce the classical picture of patches of complete hair loss and instead shows diffuse, patchy, partial hair loss. This diffuse alopecia areata can be difficult to diagnose; keep in mind the moth-

53

eaten appearance of the partial hair loss of secondary syphilis. A useful diagnostic pointer in evaluating hair loss is to look carefully for scarring: Alopecia areata doesn't scar.

Treatment

Present-day treatment of alopecia areata only temporarily modifies its course. Fortunately, most cases of alopecia areata are mild. Spontaneous hair growth frequently resumes after several months and goes on to complete regrowth. The patient information sheet has an optimistic tone since it's intended for the majority of patients for whom alopecia areata represents a passing nuisance. Do not use this sheet for a patient with severe alopecia, as the optimistic tone of the patient information sheet is inappropriate.

Is there any effective treatment? Not really. Systemic corticosteroids will almost always produce regrowth of hair in alopecia areata. However, they don't affect the ultimate result, and in patients with severe alopecia areata the new hair will promptly be shed when the corticosteroids are withdrawn. Since long-term steroids invariably produce side effects, they are not justified. True, some physicians do use systemic corticosteroids for several months in severe alopecia areata. They are not doing the patient a favor, only postponing the time when the patient must make the difficult adjustment to the hair loss.

Topical corticosteroids don't penetrate sufficiently into the skin to promote regrowth in alopecia areata. A useful approach—and often potent psychological boost—in *limited* areas of alopecia areata is the injection of repository corticosteroids. In about 75 per cent of patients hair will promptly regrow in the injected sites. Provided small amounts are injected, there's no significant systemic effect. The general technique of intralesional injection is discussed in Chapter 1. In alopecia areata I use a concentration of triamcinolone acetonide of 10 mg/ml (undiluted Kenalog 10), inject about 0.05 ml per puncture at a depth of 5 to 7 mm, and space the punctures about 1 cm apart. When injecting, be sure that the needle enters the skin at a 90° angle so as to minimize trauma and assure reproducible deposition of the corticosteroid at the necessary depth.

Inform patients that *if* the injection will stimulate hair growth, it will take about a month before that growth becomes visible. Explain that you injected a long-acting medicine that lasts three to five months (otherwise they will be on your doorstep every few weeks). I advise patients to return for further injections only if new patches of hair loss develop, and if the test injections prove effective.

Hair regrowth can be stimulated in alopecia areata by inducing skin inflammation. The inflammation must be prolonged and severe. Causing repeated bouts of contact dermatitis with dinitrochlorobenzene, a potent allergen, has been the most successful technique. Psoralen combined with ultraviolet irradiation has also been used. These approaches are still experimental, but may eventually result in a simple, practical technique.

Managing the patient

For a significant minority, the active phase of alopecia areata continues and causes extensive or recurring hair loss. Alopecia areata may extend relentlessly to complete baldness and even to loss of all body hair. In general, the earlier the onset, the worse the prognosis. Alopecia areata in young children distresses both patients and parents; in teen-agers severe alopecia areata can be an emotional disaster. Drastic personality disturbances may occur, especially in young women, since hair plays such an important role in their sexual image. Sympathetic understanding and urging these patients to wear a wig as a "temporary" measure until hair regrows may help. On occasions I've referred young patients to psychiatrists. For young persons with extensive alopecia areata, strike an optimistic note and emphasize that the hair roots are merely "resting."

Even in extensive cases when you can be fairly certain that the prognosis is bad, be optimistic. Sometimes the hair does regrow nicely, and when it doesn't, time helps patients adjust. This grim discussion applies to the *severe* cases of alopecia areata, especially when it begins in the young. Remember that in the majority of patients, events will justify your optimism.

Frequently the newly regrowing hair in alopecia areata is white rather than the color of the surrounding, unaffected hair. This color change is usually temporary but sometimes permanent. Be sympathetic; suggest that time usually corrects the color change, and encourage patients to tint their hair if they're distressed by the problem.

Basal-cell carcinoma (skin cancer) 7

Etiology

Basal-cell carcinoma is the commonest skin cancer. It results from sunlight damage to skin, although lesions aren't always located on the areas of most intense sun exposure. Basal-cell carcinoma may also occur decades after X-ray treatment. Unlike other carcinomas, basal-cell carcinoma doesn't metastasize. When informing patients they have basal-cell carcinoma, stress that it's only locally invasive and not a threat to general health. The patient instruction sheet is suitable only for basal-cell carcinoma and should not be given to patients with other skin malignancies.

Diagnosis

The appearance of the nodular basal-cell carcinoma is usually typical. It has a pearly, sharply demarcated border and shows blood vessels coursing over the surface. Sometimes there is central ulceration. Variants of basal-cell carcinoma are not so easily diagnosed; for example, superficial basal-cell carcinoma often resembles a patch of dermatitis (Figure C-13), while an infiltrating, "sclerosing" basal-cell carcinoma may resemble a scar (Figures C-8 and C-9). A tissue diagnosis is essential for proper treatment. Biopsy can be accomplished using a punch or curette or by shaving off tissue with a scissors or scalpel blade.

The chief differential diagnoses are squamous-cell carcinoma, actinic keratosis, keratoacanthoma, and such benign tumors as nevi, molluscum contagiosum, seborrheic keratosis, and warts. Watch out for the infiltrating basal-cell carcinoma, which may perfectly simulate an old scar. In this type of lesion, thin strands of tumor can infiltrate the surrounding skin without producing grossly detectable changes.

Treatment

Treatment aims to destroy the tumor with optimal cosmetic results. Surgical excision, curettage and electrodesiccation, X-ray therapy, liquid nitrogen destruction, and chemosurgery are some widely used techniques. I consider conservative surgical excision best since it provides an intact specimen for the pathologist to determine adequacy of removal, and cosmetic results are generally superior to those achieved by curettage and electrodesiccation or by irradiation.

The excision need not always be done in the standard ellipse or fusiform shape. Circular excisions using minimum 2- to 3-mm margins of normal tissue with partial closure of the defect are often useful, especially on the nose. Round lesions can be removed with a punch. The majority of basal-cell carcinomas don't penetrate significantly into the subcutaneous fat; therefore, standard conservative surgical excision usually provides adequate deep margins. The specimen should be marked on one margin—India ink works well—so that the pathologist can tell you the direction of any marginal extension of the tumor that he finds when examining step-level sections for adequacy of removal.

Ill-defined, large, or otherwise difficult lesions—especially if located near an eye or on the nose—are best treated by microscopically controlled excision (chemosurgery) (Figures C-10, C-11, and C-12). In this technique, successive planes of tissue are removed until a microscopically tumor-free plane is reached. This specialized technique, invaluable for complex cases, is now available in most major United States medical centers.

Topical chemotherapy with 5-fluorouracil for superficial basal-cell carcinomas has been advocated in advertisements. There are no guidelines as to how long to use the 5-fluorouracil, and even in experienced hands there's a significant failure rate. Leave it alone.

Complications

Recurrence and scarring are the chief complications. Careful surgical excision minimizes both these complications. Surgical excision requires more time and skill than curettage and electrodesiccation but provides superior cosmetic results.

Managing the patient

Patient education is essential. Have the patient read the basal-cell cancer information sheet and then discuss prognosis and treatment. Stress that basal-cell carcinomas do not metastasize but do require treatment, as otherwise they continue to grow relentlessly.

Follow-up is an important part of basal-cell carcinoma treatment. Traditionally, follow-up is emphasized for early detection of treatment failures. In the case of basal-cell carcinoma, follow-up turns out to be more useful for the early detection of new basal-cell carcinomas. Patients with one skin cancer are likely to develop others; of those with two or more basal-cell carcinomas, about 40 per cent will develop a new cancer within a year. Patients with skin cancers should be recalled periodically.

8

Boils (furuncles)

Etiology

Furuncles are a common skin infection caused by the ubiquitous *Staphylococcus aureus*.

Diagnosis

The most common differential diagnostic problem is distinguishing between a boil and an inflamed cyst; usually patients with inflamed cysts are aware of a preceding asymptomatic subcutaneous lump. Other bacteria and fungi occasionally produce infections resembling the staphylococcal furuncle. If you're in doubt, a gram stain and culture of pus obtained from the lesion will settle the diagnosis.

Treatment

Most boils are self-limited processes. This probably accounts for the standard textbook advice that boils need treatment only with gentle heat and possible incision and drainage if fluctuant. A minority of boils don't follow this benign, self-healing course but develop into painful abscesses or lead to burrowing and multiple carbuncle-type lesions. I find it impossible to tell which boils are going to behave aggressively, and consequently treat all early boils with systemic antibiotics. There's no point in treating a late, healing boil with systemic antibiotics since it has been walled off and systemic antibiotics won't penetrate into the infected core.

Systemic antibiotic treatment of boils should be given with the following points in mind:

1. Choose an antibiotic that's likely to be effective against staphylococci. In Western countries, most staphylococci are resistant to ordinary penicillin, tetracycline, and erythromycin. At present the drug of choice appears to be a semisynthetic, penicillinase-resistant, oral penicillin such as cloxacillin (Te-

58

gopen). In patients allergic to penicillin, clindamycin (Cleocin) and minocycline (Minocin) are reasonable alternatives.

2. If the furuncle fails to respond, or if it's located in an area of concern, e.g., near an eye, drain and aspirate the boil, culture the pus obtained, and perform sensitivity tests.

3. A five- to seven-day course of antibiotic usually suffices. The aim of the antibiotic is to stop the spread of the infection.

4. Antibiotics are not a substitute for surgical drainage if the boil contains a significant amount of pus.

Surgical drainage is indicated if pus is present or suspected. It's desirable to drain pus early, before further necrosis occurs. While the presence of fluctuation indicates pus, its absence doesn't rule out the need for surgical drainage. Furuncles, especially if deep, may have significant accumulation of pus without being fluctuant. Suspect any persistently painful boil as harboring pus in its depths.

For most boils, adequate surgical drainage can be established by a quick stab with a pointed (No. 11) blade. Refrigeration analgesia with ethyl chloride or a similar spray makes the stab more tolerable. For larger incisions, a local anesthetic should be used. It's often difficult to anesthetize a boil adequately; superficial manipulation produces deep pain because of increasing pressure on the boil.

Epinephrine should not be included in a local anesthetic used prior to minor surgery of infected tissue. There's experimental evidence in animals that the vasoconstriction produced by epinephrine encourages an infectious process to spread.

Resting the affected part is helpful, especially if the boil is on an extremity. A sling works well to immobilize the arm or hand; furuncles of the legs may require rest at home with leg elevation.

Gentle heat is part of the traditional treatment of boils; specific directions are given in the patient instruction sheet. Similarly, it's probably wise to cover draining boils with a bandage. Boils are somewhat contagious, and covering draining boils with a bandage seems a reasonable measure to minimize spread of the staphylococcus. Ask what the patient's occupation is; persons working in health-care facilities or restaurants should stay away from work until their boils have healed.

Recurrence

Recurring furunculosis is a therapeutic challenge. The majority of persons with recurring boils are otherwise healthy, although it's customary to obtain a urinalysis and blood count to rule out such underlying disorders as diabetes. It's easier to list what doesn't work for recurring furunculosis than to describe effective measures. Long-term antibiotics usually prevent new boils—provided the staphylococcus is sensitive to them. Unfortunately, in many cases boils return to plague the patient when the antibiotic is stopped. Staphylococcal vaccines have been discredited. It's difficult to assess the value of any treatment, since recurring furunculosis often lasts for many months and then disappears of its own accord.

The approach I use is to reduce the population of staphylococci on the surface of the skin and from certain areas often colonized by them. This involves applying an antimicrobial cream such as a polymyxin B-neomycin-gramicidin combination (Neosporin-G) or a chloramphenicol preparation to the nares, armpits, and groin twice daily in addition to an antiseptic over the entire skin. The antimicrobial cream to the nares, armpits, and groin is designed to eradicate staphylococci from these common reservoirs. The application of an antiseptic to the entire skin is meant to reduce the population of staphylococci on the skin. A critical number of pathogenic organisms is necessary to produce a boil.

For "degerming" the entire skin, alcohol paintings are a simple method. Seventy per cent ethyl or isopropyl alcohol is an effective antiseptic, although its action is transient. To produce a more prolonged effect, I have pharmacists prepare 0.5 per cent hexachlorophene in 70 per cent isopropyl alcohol. If there are concerns about systemic absorption of hexachlorophene, an alternative is to add benzalkonium chloride concentrate sufficient to produce a final concentration of 0.1 per cent benzalkonium chloride in 70 per cent alcohol.

9

Cysts

Etiology

Skin cysts are benign neoplasms filled with keratinous debris. Depending on the structure of the cyst wall, they are classified as epidermoid or trichilemmal. Trichilemmal cysts are commonly found on the scalp and have a tough lining that permits them to be easily shelled out. Milia (whiteheads) are small, superficial cysts. Cysts are often attached to the overlying epidermis and may communicate with the surface through a thin stalk.

Diagnosis

Diagnosis of milia and other superficial cysts is usually obvious; with deeper cysts, the diagnosis is presumptive until surgical incision. Lipomas, fibromas, and other subcutaneous tumors as well as abscesses may resemble cysts. Sebaceous-gland hyperplasia produces yellowish nodules that are distinguishable from milia by their central indentation and lobulated periphery. Chronic actinic damage may cause comedones and yellowish nodules containing small cysts and degenerated connective tissue.

Two situations present difficult differential diagnoses. The first is that of an inflamed cyst versus a furuncle. The tip-off in favor of a cyst is a history of a small, asymptomatic lump, present for months to years, that slowly enlarged until it suddenly became inflamed. Sometimes the diagnosis of inflamed cyst is made only when a "boil" is drained and fragments of cyst wall are obtained. The other differential diagnostic problem is the acne abscess, sometimes incorrectly termed "acne cyst." Acne abscesses are indolent, subcutaneous, fluctuant lesions resulting from rupture of a sebaceous gland; the resulting inflammatory response produces a pseudocapsule. Acne abscesses, unlike true cysts, don't initially possess an epithelial lining. Acne abscesses will respond to intralesional corticosteroids (Figures C-5 and C-6), whereas cysts require surgical removal of the wall. With repeated inflammation, acne abscesses may heal with formation of an epithelial lining. Patients with acne not uncommonly have both acne abscesses and true cysts.

There is no way of preventing cyst formation. Epidermoid cysts are often familial. Milia are common on the face at all ages, but are particularly a problem in elderly persons whose skin has suffered significant sun damage.

Treatment

Cysts are benign lesions; they're usually treated because the patient finds them a nuisance cosmetically or otherwise. Since a certain percentage of cysts become acutely inflamed, it may be reasonable preventive medicine to remove medium to large asymptomatic cysts. Not all subcutaneous lumps are cysts; often surgery is the only way to determine the diagnosis.

Milia are easily removed by incising the overlying skin with a small hypodermic needle (size 26 works well) and then shelling out the sac with the aid of the needle, a small, pointed splinter or jewelers' forceps, comedo extractor, and scissors. Bleeding is controlled with pressure; sutures are unnecessary. The removal site is usually invisible in two weeks. Unless the patient is stoic, I anesthetize the lesion with a drop of lidocaine and proceed at leisure, rather than have the patient squirm. Dot the milium with a felt-tipped marking pen before injecting the anesthetic, or it will be difficult to find the exact location.

Larger cysts are removed by incising the skin, dissecting out the sac, and then closing the skin with sutures. Traditionally, surgeons are taught to remove the cyst intact. This requires an incision roughly as long as the cyst. I make a small incision not more than 6 to 8 mm long and deliberately rupture the cyst sac (Figures C-14 and C-15). After the cyst contents are squeezed out, the sac is dissected away from the overlying skin with the aid of forceps, hemostat, and a small, blunt-nosed, curved scissors—a tenotomy scissors is ideal. Good lighting is essential. I prefer a head-mounted lamp and a low-power magnifying loupe. On the face and neck, linear incisions seem to work best. On the trunk, I usually incise the cyst with a 4- to 5-mm punch and dissect out the sac.

Since linear wounds on the trunk spread, slightly better cosmetic results may be obtained by starting with the small circular opening made by the punch. This is done under local anesthesia. Mark the periphery of the cyst before you anesthetize, use epinephrine with your anesthetic, and wait 15 minutes or so for maximal vasoconstriction so that you have a relatively bloodless field. The dead space resulting from the cyst is obliterated with vertical mattress sutures, which should be removed in three to five days to avoid stitch marks.

Inflamed cysts are treated by incision and drainage, accompanied by systemic antibiotics in the acute phase. The incision and drainage should be performed under local anesthesia, and the cavity scraped with a chalazion curette to remove the maximum amount of necrotic debris. Occasionally it's possible to scrape out all of the cyst wall; this relieves the immediate situation and cures the cyst. More commonly, however, some of the wall remains behind and it's necessary to excise the area after the acute inflammation has subsided. Sometimes small to medium, moderately inflamed cysts will settle down with an intralesional injection of a repository corticosteroid. These cysts should be excised later, since the corticosteroid injection doesn't destroy them.

Intralesional injection of a corticosteroid is a practical way of deciding between an acne abscess, or boil, and a cyst. If the lesion disappears, it was an acne abscess (Figures C-5 and C-6); if it doesn't, surgical treatment is indicated. Even with this precaution, one occasionally performs surgery on a presumed cyst and discovers only an acne abscess. When this happens, use a chalazion curette to scrape the cavity thoroughly, and suture the defect.

Cysts are benign; submitting a typical cyst to pathology isn't always necessary. Not infrequently one encounters a solid tumor when performing surgery on a suspected cyst. In this situation tissue examination is mandatory. If you encounter a solid tumor—usually a lipoma—try to dissect the lesion away from the surrounding tissue and deliver it intact. If you excise cysts by first rupturing the cyst wall through a tiny incision, removal of a solid tumor usually requires enlarging the incision.

The ease with which a cyst is separated from its surrounding tissue varies greatly. Trichilemmal cysts of the scalp shell out readily with pressure applied against the skull. Cysts that have undergone inflammation may adhere to the surrounding skin; they can be difficult to remove. Forget "simple" techniques of cyst destruction involving electrocoagulation of the cyst wall and overlying skin. Such measures often fail and can produce ugly scars. Unfortunately, there's no substitute for surgical removal of cysts.

Dermatitis (nonspecific dermatitis) | 10

Etiology

Dermatitis is a nonspecific reaction of the skin to a combination of exogenous and endogenous factors. It can be conveniently thought of as malfunctioning skin. Certain endogenous types of dermatitis have been classified into clinical entities: atopic eczema, psoriasis, and seborrheic dermatitis. Each is covered in a separate unit. Hand dermatitis presents special diagnostic and therapeutic problems and is discussed separately.

Dermatitis is usually a consequence of irritants, or sometimes allergens, acting on susceptible skin. The endogenous factor of susceptible skin is the most significant; often dermatitis appears without any apparent external influence. Four lines of evidence point to the usually primary role of endogenous—i.e., genetic—factors in the etiology of dermatitis:

1. Many patients with nonspecific dermatitis later develop typical atopic eczema or psoriasis.
2. A history of previous typical endogenous dermatitis, such as atopic eczema, is common.
3. A careful search often uncovers a history of dermatitis in one or more immediate blood relatives.
4. Close blood relatives of persons with eczema or psoriasis frequently develop mild, nonspecific dermatitis. This became evident to me after the siblings, parents, and children of my atopic and psoriatic patients started coming to me with similar skin complaints.

The roles of exogenous and endogenous factors are covered in Chapter 2 and are further discussed in the unit on hand dermatitis. Both patients and physicians have difficulty in accepting the significant role of endogenous factors in dermatitis; we prefer a simple cause-and-effect relationship. Dealing with the patient's concern about causes is discussed in Chapter 2. Reassure the patient that the rash is not the result of diet, "nerves," or bad health. When systemic disease is present, only in very rare instances is it related to the patient's dermatitis.

64

Diagnosis

The diagnosis of dermatitis is discussed in Chapter 2. Nonspecific dermatitis is common. Its inability to fit neatly into our clinical classifications probably accounts for the lack of textbook attention. This unit is concerned with managing the many dermatitic patients who don't have atopic dermatitis, seborrheic dermatitis, or psoriasis. Most dermatologists recognize a fourth type of dermatitis, nummular eczema (Figure C-16). Unlike the three major types of endogenous dermatitis, nummular eczema is defined only by the morphology of individual lesions. Nummular eczema consists of round patches, with minute vesicles and moderate infiltration. Lesions morphologically typical of nummular eczema can be found in many patients with classical atopic dermatitis or psoriasis. Not infrequently nummular eczema evolves into psoriasis after months or years. Because of this uncertain picture, I have chosen to lump nummular eczema with nonspecific dermatitis.

Treatment

Treatment of dermatitis boils down to:

1. Application of topical corticosteroids
2. Lubricating the skin
3. Avoiding irritants
4. Eliminating any contact allergens.

Most nonspecific dermatitis responds to the same regimen as atopic dermatitis; the majority clears up with mild or moderately potent topical corticosteroids (Chapter 1). For indurated lesions, more potent corticosteroids, possibly used with occlusion, may be necessary. Sometimes tars or intralesional corticosteroids will be required. Nummular eczema—indurated patches with tiny vesicles—often requires treatment with potent corticosteroids, tar, or both.

Skin lubrication is important. Prescribing a topical corticosteroid in a greasy ointment base is the simplest way to ensure adequate lubrication. Alternating sparing applications of white petrolatum with a corticosteroid cream, or applying white petrolatum on top of the corticosteroid cream, is also effective.

When nonspecific dermatitis is extensive, the normal skin should be lubricated to discourage the rash's further spread. Techniques for body lubrication are described in the patient dermatitis information sheet as well as the dry skin dermatitis unit.

Irritants must be avoided. Tell patients that nothing but water, their prescription medicine, and white petrolatum should touch the rash. This eliminates those common irritants, soap and over-the-counter remedies.

The most common contact allergens aggravating nonspecific dermatitis are topical medicaments. Ensuring that the patient follows your advice not to apply anything except water, the prescribed medicine, and white petrolatum virtually eliminates topical medicament allergy provided that you don't prescribe a sensitizer! Avoid prescribing neomycin, ethylenediamine (Mycolog cream), mercurials, and topical anesthetics.

Dermatitis often recurs, a point stressed in the patient information sheet. If it does, the instructions advise resuming the original treatment. Sometimes patients regard cortisone topicals as a universal remedy, good for any skin disorder. Since topical corticosteroids may actually aggravate other disorders such as impetigo and tinea pedis, the patient sheet specifically warns against using the topical drug for other skin diseases. Since potent corticosteroids may cause unpleasant side effects when used on the face or in skin-fold areas, patients are told not to apply topical corticosteroids to these areas on their own.

What if the dermatitis fails to respond?

Treatment failures are usually the result of:

1. Poor patient compliance. Have the patient describe exactly how he carries out his treatment. A useful check is to have the patient bring in the unused portion of his medication.
2. Inappropriate treatment. Use of a cream on a dry, fissured dermatitis—which needs an ointment—is a common error. Is a more potent corticosteroid indicated?
3. Irritation or allergy to a home remedy or over-the-counter medicament being used without your knowledge.
4. Irritation or allergy to the prescription medicament. The newer gel vehicles, while elegant, are often irritating. Some corticosteroid lotions, solutions, and creams contain high concentrations of propylene glycol, which may irritate the skin. Allergy to a topical medicament, while always possible, is infrequent provided the well-known sensitizers are avoided.
5. Incorrect diagnosis. Review the possibilities in Chapter 2.

Dermatitis (nonspecific)

Atopic dermatitis (atopic eczema)

11

Etiology

Atopic dermatitis, also known as atopic eczema, is a genetically determined skin disorder often affecting characteristic sites. Although significantly associated with asthma, allergic rhinitis, and urticaria, atopic dermatitis is a genetically determined disorder and not an allergic disease.

Diagnosis

Diagnosis of typical "flexural eczema" of the antecubitals and popliteals (Figure C-17) is easy. When only the face is involved, contact dermatitis—especially in a woman—is the major differential diagnosis. Contact dermatitis from an airborne agent (plants) and photosensitivity rashes may resemble atopic eczema. Atopic eczema tends to burn out with age. In later years it commonly involves only limited areas such as the face, hands, or neck. The diagnostic tip-off is a history of atopic dermatitis in infancy or childhood. A family history of atopic dermatitis is also significant.

Atopic dermatitis in the infant usually doesn't show the typical flexural localization. It tends to be more diffuse and involve the trunk, face, and extremities. It may be difficult to distinguish infantile atopic dermatitis from seborrheic dermatitis. Sometimes the family history is more helpful than the morphology of the eruption in the differential diagnosis. While the treatment of most endogenous dermatoses in infancy is similar—essentially topical corticosteroids—the prognosis is different. Infantile seborrheic dermatitis usually disappears within a year or two, while atopic dermatitis is often a chronic process.

The tendency of eczema of infants and children to clear spontaneously with age is well known. But be cautious about reassuring parents that their infant will soon outgrow his atopic eczema. In many cases eczema continues—sometimes intermittently clearing—into adulthood. The atopic diathesis is still present in these adults, and frequently manifests itself in later life in the form of localized eczema favoring the hands, neck, genital area, and face.

Sometimes such localized atopic dermatitis resembles psoriasis or the lichenified chronic localized dermatitis described as lichen simplex chronicus.

Complications

In the majority of cases, atopic eczema is a nuisance readily controllable by topical measures. Cataracts are an occasional complication of severe atopic eczema. Atopic patients—especially infants and young children—are prone to secondary infection. A justly feared complication of atopic eczema is generalized infection with herpes simplex or vaccinia virus. Formerly called Kaposi's varicelliform eruption, it's now referred to as either eczema herpeticum or eczema vaccinatum. Since smallpox vaccination has been abandoned, the herpes simplex virus is now the cause of this eruption. Eczema herpeticum can be a serious medical complication requiring specialized hospital care.

Two popular misconceptions about atopic dermatitis

Two widely held misconceptions interfere with the rational therapy of eczema. The first is that atopic eczema is an allergic diathesis requiring extensive (and expensive) diagnostic skin tests and therapy with dietary restriction and desensitization injections. Neither treatment is of value. Physicians treating atopic eczema with desensitization and diet therapy almost invariably prescribe topical corticosteroids as an "adjunct." Since more than 90 per cent of atopic eczemas clear nicely with corticosteroids alone, the pointlessness of desensitization therapy is evident.

Dietary therapy is of no value in adult atopic eczema. I have yet to see an adult with atopic eczema whose rash consistently flared up when he consumed certain foods. Food allergy occasionally complicates atopic eczema in infants and children. Eggs, sometimes milk, and rarely wheat can be offenders. When infantile atopic eczema fails to repond to topical management, have the parents eliminate eggs and milk for three or four weeks. If the eczema improves significantly, the child should be fed large "challenge" amounts of the suspected food to see if the eczema flares up. If it does, the elimination and challenge should be repeated once to make sure these weren't chance events—atopic eczema is prone to spontaneous remissions and flare-ups. Elimination-diet trials should be limited to three or four weeks, and diet elimination continued thereafter only if a causal effect can be demonstrated. One occasionally encounters malnourished youngsters as a result of ill-advised, unnecessarily prolonged elimination diets.

The second common misconception is that atopic eczema is a nervous disorder or "neurodermatitis" to be treated by psychotherapy or with tranquilizers or sedatives. This is cruel and inept: cruel because the patient is unjustly blamed for his "nerves" causing the eczema, and inept because it leads to inappropriate therapy with tranquilizers and sedatives. This is not to say that emotional upsets play no role in atopic eczema; they frequently worsen it. Furthermore, a significant number of atopic patients—like a significant number of the general population—have emotional disorders warranting psychotherapy. Atopic eczema is not a conversion reaction and needs appropriate dermatologic treatment, not psychotherapy. Sedatives and tranquilizers will make an itching patient more comfortable by dulling his sensorium; it's preferable to suppress the underlying skin disease.

Treatment

Topical therapy

Topical corticosteroids will effectively control atopic eczema in well over 90 per cent of patients (Figures C-17 and C-18). Their use is discussed in Chapter 1. Keep in mind that (1) significant systemic absorption may occur when large areas of eczematous skin are treated with topical corticosteroids and (2) fluorinated corticosteroids should not be used on the face or skin-fold areas. Show patients how to apply the corticosteroid and give them the "Cortisone Ointments" instruction sheet.

If topical corticosteroids fail to provide adequate control, add coal tar to the regimen. A tar-oil bath additive produces a mild tar effect. Crude-coal-tar-containing lotions, creams, gels, or ointments applied thinly at bedtime achieve a more potent tar effect. Details of the use of coal-tar preparations are given in the unit on psoriasis.

Coal tar is irritating to some persons and occasionally sensitizes, causing contact dermatitis. It's best to initiate coal-tar therapy by having the patient apply it to only a small area for one week as a therapeutic trial.

Other topical agents are best avoided. Topical antimicrobials are generally unnecessary; if there's significant secondary infection, it should be treated with oral antibiotics.

Patients frequently aggravate their dermatitis with inappropriate self-treatment. Instruct your patients not to apply anything to their skin except as you direct. Clinically it's difficult to distinguish a spontaneous flare-up of atopic eczema from eczema aggravated by irritation or allergic contact dermatitis. Consequently, try to exclude the likelihood that a topical medicament is aggravating the eczema.

Hand dermatitis as part of atopic eczema may be a stubborn problem. Treat hand dermatitis according to its severity as outlined in the next unit.

Intralesional corticosteroids

Intralesional injection of repository corticosteroids is a neat way of treating stubborn, localized atopic eczema. The technique is described in Chapter 1.

Systemic therapy

Systemic corticosteroids are occasionally necessary for severe atopic eczema. Usually a one- to two-week course will suffice. Use prednisone given as a single morning dose. Begin with enough—usually 60 to 80 mg a day for an adult—and decrease the dosage by 5 to 10 mg a day as soon as improvement occurs. The aim of systemic corticosteroids is to relieve the inflammation and swelling to a point where topical steroids can control it. If proper topical therapy is initiated, it will rarely be necessary to use systemic corticosteroids for more than two weeks. If more than two weeks of systemic corticosteroids are required, the patient should be switched to every-other-day prednisone and weaned off it gradually. When prolonged systemic corticosteroids are required to control atopic eczema, search for a complicating contact dermatitis. Sometimes what appears to be recalcitrant atopic eczema is actually atopic eczema that is complicated by contact dermatitis, usually caused by a topical medicament.

Systemic antibiotics are indicated when atopic eczema becomes infected, a not uncommon occurrence. I prefer either erythromycin or an oral semisynthetic penicillin such as cloxacillin (Tegopen). A five- to eight-day course usually suffices. It's sometimes difficult to know whether oozing and crusting are part of the eczematous process or represent secondary infection. A gram-stained smear of intact pustules is a more reliable test for infection than a culture. Cultures may be misleading, since dermatitic skin is frequently colonized by pathogenic bacteria without resultant disease. Cultures can't distinguish between colonization and infection. Clinical judgment is usually reliable; if you're in doubt, there's little harm in a short course of oral antibiotic.

Other measures

Patients with eczema invariably have dry skin. They will benefit from systematic lubrication (Figures C-17 and C-18) as explained in the dry-skin dermatitis instruction sheet. Stress that they are to use only the lubricants and procedures that you recommend.

Atopic eczema is frequently worsened by nervous tension, contact with rough woolen clothing, cold weather, or extremely hot weather. Stress and nervous tension are part and parcel of life; however, the other aggravating factors can be avoided or minimized. Woolen garments should not be worn next to the skin; this also holds true for any roughly textured synthetic fabric. The deleterious effect of wool on atopic skin results from mechanical irritation, not allergy.

Cold weather, with its low humidity, desiccates atopic skin and leads to fissuring and dermatitis. To counteract this drying effect, have patients lubricate their skins more frequently and intensively during winter. The use of humidifiers at home may help.

Hot weather is notorious for producing severe atopic flare-ups. Sweating is defective in dermatitic skin, so tell the patient to avoid severe heat stress. Air conditioning is the appropriate remedy. If only one room can be air-conditioned, it should be the bedroom.

Atopic dermatitis

12

Hand dermatitis

Hand dermatitis is common. It causes patients a great deal of anguish, may be seriously disabling, and is frustrating to physicians. The classical method of dermatologic diagnosis—evaluating morphology and distribution of the rash—often fails in hand dermatitis. Most hand eczemas (the words *eczema* and *dermatitis* are used interchangeably) tend to look alike even though their etiologies differ. Hand eczema is often chronic; what doctor hasn't shuddered on seeing a new patient whose hand eczema has plagued her for years while she made the rounds of local physicians? Hand eczema is a clinical entity in its own right. While there is often hand involvement in atopic dermatitis or psoriasis, we don't speak of it as hand eczema, but rather as atopic dermatitis or psoriasis of the hands (see Figures C-31 and C-32). Usually the cause of hand eczema isn't obvious. Most hand dermatoses are the result of nonspecific irritation in a person predisposed to develop dermatitis. Fortunately, the therapy of nonspecific hand dermatitis is the same as for atopic or psoriatic hand dermatitis.

There is a rational way to approach the diagnosis of hand dermatitis. Furthermore, most hand eczemas do well with topical corticosteroids, systematic lubrication, and avoidance of irritants. Successful treatment hinges on using measures appropriate to the site and severity of the dermatitis. Both treatment and hand protection require meticulous attention to detail; the printed instruction forms are invaluable in managing hand dermatitis.

Don't let the length of this unit turn you off. The majority of patients with hand dermatitis do well when provided with proper advice and a topical corticosteroid. Precise treatment directions are given in the sheet titled "Hand Dermatitis Treatment," while general care of the hands is detailed in the hand protection sheet. If you prefer to treat only mild hand dermatitis and refer the severe cases, proceed to the topical therapy instructions.

Those wishing to wrestle with the more difficult hand dermatoses should study the sections on etiology and diagnosis. Severe hand dermatitis, while relatively infrequent, is a major therapeutic headache. Its successful treatment requires scrupulous attention to details, and the necessary information cannot be condensed.

Etiology

Hand dermatitis results from the skin's inability to cope with local noxious influences. To varying degrees endogenous and exogenous factors are involved in its causation. These factors, summarized in Table 12-1, interact in subtle and complex ways; for discussion purposes they're treated separately.

Endogenous factors

Atopic dermatitis

Atopic dermatitis frequently involves the hands. Only the hands may be involved in an adult or teen-ager who had typical flexural atopic eczema as a small child. A history of previous atopic eczema in a person with hand dermatitis is strong evidence for its being atopic hand eczema. A history of atopic dermatitis in close relatives suggests that atopic factors may be significant in producing the dermatitis.

Psoriasis

Psoriasis causes many chronic cases of hand dermatitis (see Figures C-31 and C-32). There may be little or no psoriatic involvement elsewhere. In many cases involvement of the soles and/or perianal area or a plaque on the scalp will tell you that you're dealing with psoriasis. Psoriasis in close blood relatives should alert you to consider psoriasis as a possible cause.

Psoriasiform disorders

There are several curious disorders affecting the hands and/or feet and characterized by recurring grouped vesicles or pustules and a chronic course. The pustules are sterile. Dermatologists don't agree on their nomenclature;

TABLE 12-1

Endogenous and exogenous factors involved in hand dermatitis

Endogenous
Atopic dermatitis
Psoriasis
Psoriasiform disorders
   Vesiculopustular disorders of hands, i.e., dyshidrosis, pompholyx, acral pustulosis, pustular bacterid, pustulosis palmaris et plantaris, etc.
Nummular eczema

Exogenous
Irritants: acids, alkalies, soaps, detergents, solvents, etc.
Allergens (contact allergy): vast number of possible allergens; of particular significance in chronic hand dermatitis are topical medicaments

Reprinted, with permission, from *Cutis* 15:346, 1975.

Hand dermatitis

they're varyingly diagnosed as dyshidrosis, pustulosis palmaris et plantaris, acral pustulosis, pustular bacterid, or acrovesiculatio recidivans. These psoriasiform disorders are suppressed by corticosteroids—and not much else. In many such cases there's psoriasis on some part of the body. I group these conditions together because they respond similarly to treatment.

Exogenous factors

Irritants

Irritants such as acids, strong alkalies, and detergents act nonspecifically to inflame skin. We're all exposed to irritants, but we don't all have hand dermatitis. One factor is the level of exposure to irritants; more housewives, waiters, and nurses, for example, have hand eczema than do accountants. Because endogenous factors are also significant, not all housewives have hand eczema. Irritants aggravate any hand dermatitis, irrespective of underlying causes, and must be carefully avoided. Irritants are the most important exogenous causes of hand dermatitis.

Allergens (contact allergy)

Allergic contact dermatitis can either be a primary cause of hand dermatitis or aggravate a pre-existing hand eczema. In a few cases, contact allergy is the sole cause of hand dermatitis. It's important to ferret out these cases; they are curable. In industrial workers the chance that a specific allergen is the cause of dermatitis must be carefully considered. This is especially true for certain occupations, such as cement workers, since cement allergy is a common cause of hand dermatitis. A careful inquiry as to the nature of the work, substances encountered at work, and relationship of the dermatitis to vacation periods should be made. Pinpointing the specific contactant requires patch testing by a specialist, since reliable patch testing with industrial materials is difficult. In housewives, contact allergy is rarely the primary cause of hand dermatitis.

IMPORTANT: In men and women with hand dermatitis of varying etiologies, 10 to 20 per cent have superimposed contact dermatitis from a topical medicament used to treat the primary rash.

Making the diagnosis

The steps in diagnosing hand eczema are outlined in Table 12-2. First, search for endogenous factors by inquiring about a past history of eczema, especially atopic eczema in infancy and childhood. Do close blood relatives have hand eczema, psoriasis, or other chronic skin problems? A commonly seen pattern, especially in women, is that of atopic eczema in infancy that clears up in childhood only to recur as hand eczema in the teens or 20s.

Note whether the rash is primarily volar or dorsal. Hand dermatitis limited to the palms is usually endogenous. The dorsal skin is more sensitive to external irritants or allergens and is usually involved when exogenous factors are significant. Symmetry—especially if only the palms are involved—

TABLE 12-2

Diagnostic steps in evaluation of chronic hand dermatitis

History
Occupation and time relationship to work
Effect of vacations
Family history of hand eczema, dermatitis, psoriasis, or eczema
Previous and current topical therapy
    Chemicals, medicaments, lubricating creams, rubber gloves applied to hands or currently used at work, home, or in hobbies

Examination
Hands
    Dorsal versus volar involvement
    Nail pitting with normal paronychial tissues
    Vesicles or pustules of palms
General
    Examine the entire skin! Feet and perianal skin are especially important

Reprinted, with permission, from *Cutis* 15:346, 1975.

also favors endogenous causes. These are guidelines, not absolute rules.

Look carefully at the nails. Pits or marked dystrophic changes with normal cuticles are good evidence of psoriasis. If the posterior nail fold is involved in dermatitis, the nails will show dystrophic changes irrespective of the cause of hand dermatitis; that's why pitting is significant only when the nail folds are normal.

Examine the patient's entire skin, paying particular attention to the feet and perianal area. Dermatitis on other parts of the body is strong evidence of an endogenous component of the hand eczema. Often the only evidence of a psoriatic factor in hand dermatitis is typical psoriasis involving the perianal skin and gluteal cleft (Figures C-33, C-34, and C-35). Many patients deny having any rash other than on their hands—only to have the examination contradict their statement. Look carefully at the feet. If the feet and hands both have dermatitis, this is strong evidence of an endogenous cause.

Exogenous factors

The two most important areas of questioning are (1) the patient's occupation and (2) what the patient has been applying to his hands as lubricants and medication. Persons with certain occupations, such as housewives, dishwashers, or waitresses, are heavily exposed to irritants and encounter relatively few potential allergens. In other occupations one must think of an allergen as a possible cause, especially if the patient handles such well-known allergens as epoxy glues, chromate-containing materials, or formaldehyde. What happens to his rash when he goes on vacation? If there is strong suspi-

Hand dermatitis

cion of an occupational allergen, the patient should be referred to a specialist experienced in patch testing. Don't attempt patch testing unless you've had special training in it; otherwise errors of execution and interpretation of the patch test are likely.

Previously used lotions, creams, and medicaments—both over-the-counter and prescription—frequently aggravate hand dermatitis. Have the patient list everything he has been applying to his hands and ask him to bring in all his topical medicaments at the next visit. You may be surprised at the number (and nature) of topicals employed, and how many he forgot to mention when you took his history.

These steps will give you an idea of the respective roles of endogenous and exogenous factors and help you formulate treatment. Conversely, the treatment results will influence your diagnosis. Most hand dermatoses clear rapidly with treatment and don't require sophisticated investigation. On the other hand, a recalcitrant process may require repeated, detailed questioning as to contactants, a variety of therapeutic approaches, and, possibly, patch testing.

Differential diagnosis

The catch-all label of hand eczema is usually appropriately applied by most physicians. There is one disorder that occasionally traps even the wary—tinea manum. Tinea manum is frequently unilateral, affects mainly the palms, and is sharply demarcated; frequently there are dystrophic changes in one or more fingernails. The feet invariably have tinea pedis, but this isn't particularly helpful as tinea pedis is common in the general population. Finding the organism on KOH-cleared scrapings, or on culture, is diagnostic; you won't find it unless you suspect a fungus and look for it. Griseofulvin (Fulvicin, Grifulvin, Grisactin) or ketoconazole (Nizoral) by mouth promptly clears this disorder, although it usually relapses.

Bowen's disease (intraepidermal squamous-cell carcinoma) often looks like eczema. Its unchanging nature and failure to respond to treatment should lead to biopsy and the correct diagnosis. Other disorders, such as lichen planus, drug eruptions, and subacute lupus erythematosus, may involve the hands. Usually these processes involve other parts of the body in addition to the hands; examination of the entire skin may point toward the correct diagnosis.

The trichophytid, or "id," reaction on the fingers associated with fungus of the feet is a definite entity, but not as common as was formerly thought. An "id" hand eruption is a hypersensitivity process triggered by tinea pedis. Before griseofulvin, it was a commonly given explanation for vesicular eruptions of the fingers and palms. The "id" reaction is rarely the sole cause of a hand eruption. Only occasionally is it possible to clear a hand eruption by vigorous treatment of tinea pedis with internal griseofulvin and the newer topical fungicides. Most patients previously diagnosed as having "ids" have chronic vesicular hand eruptions that are aggravated in a nonspecific way by activation of their tinea pedis.

Treatment

Eliminating causes

Two aims should be kept in mind in managing hand dermatitis: (1) elimination of the cause(s) and (2) suppression of the dermatitis with active therapy.

Eliminating the cause(s) is more easily said than done; usually there are multiple causes, only some of which can be altered. Endogenous factors—a constitutional tendency toward eczema—cannot be changed. Of the exogenous factors, irritants are the most common. Systematic protection of the hands is essential. Every patient with hand dermatitis should be given the hand protection instruction sheet—but don't stop there. Go over the significant points, and ask the patient to read the instructions daily for a week. For many patients, such as housewives, nurses, or dishwashers, it will be impossible to follow the hand protection instructions precisely. Stress that they are a goal to be aimed at. Over-the-counter hand creams and lotions and various self-treatment routines are frequently irritating; insist that the patient apply only what you have prescribed.

It's harder to eliminate contact with possible allergens than to avoid irritants; irritants are usually easily identified. The most commonly identified allergen aggravating hand dermatitis is a topical medicament. Benzocaine and other topical anesthetics, mercurial antimicrobials, and neomycin and ethylenediamine (Mycolog cream) are common offenders. Don't prescribe these preparations; be sure the patient isn't using any such product he bought over the counter, obtained from a friend, or received from a previous physician.

Eliminating contact with other possible environmental allergens is a challenge. One has to establish that the patient has a relevant contact allergy—that he's allergic to something his hands touch. This can entail prolonged, involved studies; fortunately, they're rarely necessary. The vast majority of hand dermatoses do nicely with careful hand protection and appropriate topical therapy and do not require patch testing.

This is to stress again that in treating hand dermatitis, therapy does not simply follow diagnosis; there should be continuing interaction, for diagnosis is influenced by the response to treatment. The common housewife's hand dermatitis usually responds well to protective routines and topical corticosteroids. When it does, it's assumed to be basically an irritant process. When a hand dermatitis doesn't respond to therapy, a continuing search for causes should be undertaken. Sometimes only prolonged observation clarifies the diagnosis. This is especially the case in psoriasis of the hands, which may begin insidiously as a nonspecific-appearing hand dermatitis.

Active therapy

Active therapy can be summarized in one word: corticosteroids. In spite of the bewildering array of diagnostic designations applied to hand dermatitis—atopic eczema, housewife's hand dermatitis, pustulosis palmaris, dyshidrosis, pompholyx, nummular eczema, psoriasis of the palms—they all respond to corticosteroids and virtually nothing else. The discussion will be restricted to the use of corticosteroids and will reflect the severity and location of the dermatitis rather than esoteric diagnostic terms. As most hand dermatoses require prolonged therapy, the emphasis will be on topical corticosteroids. Result: Treating hand dermatitis is simple, safe, and rewarding.

Systemic corticosteroids

In the acute, severe, blistering hand dermatitis a brief course of systemic corticosteroids gives dramatic benefit. The aim of the systemic drug is to render the dermatitis susceptible to topical corticosteroids; when there is edema and blistering, topical corticosteroids won't penetrate deeply enough to be effective. Usually a four- to seven-day tapering course of steroid suffices. Prednisone is the drug of choice, given as one dose in the morning. Since you'll use systemic corticosteroids only for severe processes, prescribe enough: 60 to 80 mg of prednisone the first day, decreased by 10 to 20 mg each day thereafter. Begin topical corticosteroid therapy when there is some decrease in blistering and swelling.

Avoid systemic therapy with injections of long-acting repository corticosteroids such as triamcinolone acetonide. Not only do they cause prolonged adrenal suppression, but the patient observes that for the next few weeks his hands do well no matter what he does. He never learns the technique or the effectiveness of proper topical therapy. When three to six weeks later the hand eczema flares, he returns for another "magic" shot.

Other systemic therapies

When bacterial infection is present or suspected, systemic antibiotics are indicated; either erythromycin or a semisynthetic penicillin (such as cloxacillin) taken by mouth. In the presence of hand infection, it's preferable to prescribe a systemic antibiotic and a topical corticosteroid rather than rely on topical applications of an antibiotic-corticosteroid combination.

Mentioned only to be condemned are antihistamines, sedatives, and tranquilizers. They do not improve dermatitis, but only dull the patient's sensorium. There are always rare exceptions; a highly anxious patient may need a few days of support with a tranquilizer or mild sedative taken at bedtime.

Topical therapy

General principles

Topical corticosteroids are the essence, mainstay, and sheet anchor (choose your favorite noun) of treating hand dermatitis. The only time they are not of value is in the initial stages of an acute dermatitis with blisters and marked edema. Topical adjuncts are cool tap-water soaks and lubrication as needed with sparing applications of white petrolatum.

The choice of topical corticosteroid therapy depends on the location and severity of the dermatitis. Dermatitis of the backs of the hands responds much more readily to topical corticosteroids than does palmar dermatitis. The effectiveness of topical therapy can be increased both by using more potent steroids and by plastic occlusion. Plastic occlusion increases corticosteroid penetration roughly 10 times. If there is significant volar dermatitis, plastic occlusion will usually be required.

Plastic occlusion increases the unwanted as well as the desirable effects of corticosteroids. The fluorinated formulations may cause skin atrophy; plastic occlusion markedly accentuates it. Clinically such atrophy appears as thin, irritated skin with easy fissuring. The patient usually complains of sensitive, easily injured skin. Sometimes atrophy is mistaken for a flare-up of the dermatitis and is made worse by more vigorous treatment with high-potency corticosteroids.

Occlusion of the hands is best accomplished by wearing thin, pliable, properly fitting plastic (*not* rubber) gloves overnight. It's uncomfortable, but after a few days the benefits become so obvious that patients usually cease their complaints. Be sure the gloves aren't too tight; fit the patient with the proper size and hand him one or two pairs for extras. The brand is unimportant, but it is important that the gloves be pliable, slightly elastic, and readily available.

To avoid atrophy, use the minimum amount of occlusion and the least potent corticosteroid needed to control the dermatitis. For long-term use 1 per cent hydrocortisone is best, as it doesn't cause hand skin atrophy. Patients vary greatly in their tolerance of fluorinated corticosteroids; while some tolerate them for years, others show undesirable atrophy after a few weeks of use (see Figure C-32). Hand dermatitis treatment should be tailored to location and severity to produce adequate suppression with minimal risk of atrophy.

This system of managing hand dermatitis centers about a treatment instruction sheet that provides precise directions for the use of topical corticosteroids. This basic instruction sheet is given to all hand dermatitis patients; the physician chooses the topical corticosteroid appropriate to the severity of the patient's dermatitis.

For patients with severe or volar hand dermatitis, the basic hand treatment routine is supplemented by overnight plastic occlusion. The technique and its side effects are described in the instruction sheet "Overnight Plastic Occlusion for Hand Dermatitis." When the basic hand dermatitis treatment is supplemented by overnight occlusion, the physician should prescribe either two topical corticosteroids or a potent corticosteroid plus a lubricant. A small amount of moderate- to high-potency corticosteroid will be required for bedtime applications before the patient puts on the plastic gloves. During the day the patient uses either a bland emollient or an inexpensive, low-potency corticosteroid for lubrication.

To summarize: After history and examination,

1. Provide the hand dermatitis treatment sheet.
2. Provide the hand protection instructions.
3. Briefly go over the instructions and tell the patient to read both sheets daily for a week to fix them in his mind.
4. Write a prescription for a topical corticosteroid.

Simple, and it works. For mild dermatitis prescribe a low-potency corticosteroid; for moderate dermatitis, a stronger one. For severe dermatitis—especially if there's volar involvement—plastic occlusion should be used overnight. If you don't want to get involved with occlusion and high-potency corticosteroids, stick to treating mild or moderate dorsal dermatitis and refer severer cases.

Specific details

Mild dorsal dermatitis. The majority of hand dermatoses seen in housewives and others exposed to heavy use of irritants show mainly dorsal involvement; erythema and scaling dominate. Occlusion isn't needed. Prescribe 1 per cent hydrocortisone cream or a low-potency fluorinated corticosteroid. The patient should apply the topical thinly to the entire skin of both hands— like a hand cream—and use it many times a day.

Often creams are not lubricating enough but ointments are too greasy. That's why the patient is given the option of applying plain white petrolatum after the corticosteroid cream. An alternative approach (and one that I prefer) is to have the pharmacist add 15 to 25 per cent white petrolatum to the corticosteroid cream.

Have the pharmacist put up the prescription in two jars. Housewives should keep one jar in the kitchen, the other in the bathroom, for frequent use after hand washing. For those working outside the home, one container should be kept at work.

The patient returns in one to two weeks. If you're on the right track, there will be dramatic improvement. Go over the long-term aspects of treatment and specifically explain to the patient how to reduce the frequency of application gradually. If the patient was originally given a fluorinated corticosteroid, I usually shift him to a 1 per cent hydrocortisone topical for maintenance. While most patients' hands tolerate long-term use of low-potency fluorinated corticosteroids without occlusion, atrophy occurs in some.

Moderate dorsal dermatitis. In moderately severe dorsal dermatitis I use a highly potent corticosteroid once or twice a day with*out* occlusion. A bland lubricant or 1 per cent hydrocortisone cream is used frequently during the day. As the patient improves, the potent corticosteroid is gradually phased out. This approach requires two minor changes in the printed directions. Cross out "cortisone medicine" in the first sentence and substitute "special lubricant" or the name of an over-the-counter preparation. At the bottom add a sentence directing the patient to apply the highly potent corticosteroid sparingly to the rash area at bedtime.

When the dermatitis has cleared, the patient continues the lubricating treatment on a long-term basis. Recurring dermatitis is an indication for resuming nightly use of the high-potency corticosteroid.

If a highly potent corticosteroid is applied once daily, either with or without occlusion, it makes little difference whether 1 per cent hydrocortisone or a bland emollient is used for skin lubrication. The potent corticosteroid completely overshadows any effect of the hydrocortisone. Nevertheless, my preference is to use 1 per cent hydrocortisone cream (often with 15 to 25 per cent petrolatum) as a basic skin lubricant even when a highly potent corticosteroid is used simultaneously. After the high-potency corticosteroid has been phased out, the hydrocortisone-containing lubricant usually controls recurrences. Treatment is simplified, since the patient uses only one preparation—his hydrocortisone topical—to control minor flare-ups. This regimen is a personal preference, unsupported by controlled studies.

Hand dermatitis with significant volar involvement. When there is significant involvement of volar surfaces and/or severe dermatitis of the dorsa, overnight occlusion should be added initially to frequent daytime corticosteroid or lubricant applications. The overnight occlusion should be considered a "booster" treatment. For the overnight occlusion only, a moderate- to high-potency corticosteroid should be employed. The daytime medication should be a bland emollient or an inexpensive hydrocortisone preparation, since the patient will use it as a lubricant.

Depending on severity, for occlusion treatment use either a moderate- or high-potency fluorinated corticosteroid or 3 to 6 per cent hydrocortisone in white petrolatum. Stress that the occlusion should be confined to the rash and not used on the entire hand. If the eruption is limited to the palms, cut the fingers off the plastic gloves. When the dermatitis involves only fingers, the patient is to cut the appropriate fingers off the plastic glove and hold them in place overnight with nonirritating "paper" tape.

Have the patient return 7 to 10 days after initiating treatment; if he's better, ask him to use occlusion only every other night. If he does well on every-other-night occlusion, instruct him at the next visit to use it only every third night; after an additional two weeks, see if he can discontinue occlusion. Back away from overnight occlusion when the dermatitis is better, and before clinically obvious atrophy occurs. With care, this can usually be done. IMPORTANT: Provide only a small amount of high-potency corticosteroid so the patient can't continue treatment for months on his own.

Most patients can be weaned away from occlusion, although some find it necessary to use it once or twice a week indefinitely. Long-term occlusive treatment with a potent corticosteroid is usually safe when used not more than twice a week. It may be possible to shift the patient to hydrocortisone or an intermediate-strength fluorinated corticosteroid, with occasional occlusion as the situation demands.

Variations

These treatment methods can and should be modified. Volar dermatitis affecting only the fingers frequently responds to nightly use of a high-potency corticosteroid without occlusion. Patients who object to overnight occlusion may successfully treat their hands by wearing the plastic gloves for three or four hours while awake. If the patient objects to petrolatum as a lubricant, prescribe something less greasy. Be willing to modify your treatment to fit your patients; the medicament or lubricant will work only if they comply with the treatment program.

Hand dermatitis

Intralesional therapy

Intralesional corticosteroids are useful in hand dermatitis when there's a small but active area of dermatitis and when there's extensive vesicular volar dermatitis that responds poorly to occlusion with potent corticosteroids. The technique and problems of intralesional therapy are described in Chapter 1. Intralesional corticosteroid injections into the hands should be used reluctantly, as infection occasionally follows.

Seborrheic dermatitis

13

Etiology

This common skin disorder is misnamed, for seborrheic dermatitis has nothing to do with the sebaceous glands. It's a genetically determined skin dysfunction; the mechanism is unknown.

Diagnosis

Typical cases are easily diagnosed since seborrheic dermatitis commonly favors (1) the scalp and scalp margins, (2) the glabella, eyebrows, and eyelid edges, (3) the skin about the nose, (4) the ears and retroauricular folds, (5) the presternal area and mid-upper back, and (6) skin folds—inguinal, gluteal, axillary, and inframammary.

The scalp is the commonest location; ordinary dandruff* is seborrheic dermatitis of the scalp. Frequently the rash spreads onto the forehead and lateral scalp margins. The rash of seborrheic dermatitis is red and scaly except in skin-fold areas, where it usually takes on a smooth, red, glazed appearance.

Psoriasis is the chief differential diagnosis. On the scalp seborrheic dermatitis tends to form diffuse, scaling areas with mild redness, while psoriasis shows sharply demarcated, infiltrated, often crusted plaques. Frequently it's impossible to be sure what disease is present, and some physicians express their diagnostic uncertainty by using the term *seborrhiasis*. Not uncommonly a patient will have typical seborrheic dermatitis of the scalp that gradually worsens over the years, becomes recalcitrant to therapy, and finally presents as typical psoriasis.

In skin-fold areas, seborrheic dermatitis and psoriasis frequently have the same red, glazed appearance. Candidiasis and dermatophytosis (tinea cruris)

---

*An oversimplification. The current view is that mild, noninflammatory dandruff represents the physiologic desquamation of the scalp known as pityriasis capitis. Patients with "dandruff" show a spectrum of severity of scalp scaling. In mild cases it's usually impossible to decide whether the process should be considered physiologic (pityriasis capitis) or a mild form of disease (seborrheic dermatitis). From a practical viewpoint, such considerations are immaterial; the treatment of pityriasis capitis is the same as that of mild seborrheic dermatitis.

must be differentiated and can sometimes coexist with seborrheic dermatitis. Stubborn diaper rash is usually seborrheic dermatitis, sometimes with superimposed candidiasis and frequently with irritation from topical therapy. Cradle cap is seborrheic dermatitis of the scalp in infants.

Always keep psoriasis in the back of your mind when managing patients with seborrheic dermatitis.

Treatment

At the outset, be sure your patient understands that treatment is a matter of control rather than cure. Failure to accept this will invariably lead to dissatisfaction. While seborrheic dermatitis is a chronic, recurring condition, it usually responds nicely to topical therapy. Secondary infection—manifested by oozing, pustules, and crusting—occurs occasionally, especially about the ears. A five- to seven-day course of erythromycin or a semisynthetic penicillin by mouth generally clears this. Systemic corticosteroids are not indicated unless there's a superimposed severe contact dermatitis.

Corticosteroids, tars, sulfur, and salicylic acid are the preferred topicals. I consider iodochlorhydroxyquin (Vioform) to be outmoded, as it stains clothes and occasionally sensitizes. Treatment of seborrheic dermatitis depends on its site as well as its severity, and therefore will be discussed in this chapter on a regional basis.

Scalp

Mild dandruff is most easily controlled by frequent shampooing. Ask the patient to shampoo, if practical, whenever he showers. The type of shampoo used is less critical than the frequency of shampooing. Treatment routines are somewhat arbitrary. My favorite approach is to have the patient shampoo once every two weeks with 2.5 per cent selenium sulfide shampoo (a prescription item) and in between shampoo as often as possible with a tar or other "medicated" over-the-counter shampoo. If you have samples, have the patient try them and pick his favorite. Stress that daily shampooing is safe and does not cause hair loss (a common misconception).

If frequent medicated shampoos fail to control scalp seborrhea, topical corticosteroids or tars are indicated. It's more difficult to deliver medications to the hairy scalp than to smooth skin. Creams and ointments are out. For moderate seborrheic dermatitis, prescribe a corticosteroid gel or liquid to be applied sparingly once daily and massaged in well. These are clean, elegant preparations that neither stink nor stain.

Tars are the next step if frequent shampooing and a topical corticosteroid fail to provide adequate control. A coal-tar gel (Psorigel, Estar Gel) can be massaged in sparingly three to eight hours before shampooing, or, as an alternative, a tar-oil bath additive (Balnetar) can be painted sparingly on the scaly areas three to eight hours before shampooing. Warn patients that tars can photosensitize and cause sunburning of the scalp.

If the combination of frequent shampoos, a topical corticosteroid, and a tar applied before shampooing fail to control seborrheic dermatitis, the patient almost certainly has psoriasis.

Ears and scalp edges

A fluorinated corticosteroid in gel, cream, or ointment form applied once or twice daily usually produces dramatic control. Write on the prescription, and also instruct the patient, that the medication must not be used on the face. For the scalp edges, gels and lotions are preferable. On the ears, a greasy corticosteroid ointment applied just at bedtime is usually very effective.

Face

One per cent hydrocortisone cream applied thinly two to four times daily and massaged in well will control most seborrheic dermatitis of the face. Do not use fluorinated corticosteroids on the face. If 1 per cent hydrocortisone cream is inadequate, add 2 per cent sulfur and 2 per cent salicylic acid to the hydrocortisone cream. If control is still inadequate, increase the hydrocortisone strength to 2 to 3 per cent, possibly with added sulfur and salicylic acid, each at 2 per cent.

Eyelids

Seborrheic blepharitis with its crusting and itching eyelid edges is a common chronic problem. Eyelid crusting often responds to diluted Johnson's baby shampoo (*no* other brand) applied to the edges of the lids with a cotton-tipped swab. Ophthalmologists are fond of treating seborrheic blepharitis with topical antimicrobials such as sulfacetamide ointment. In my experience, an antibiotic-hydrocortisone ointment combination is superior to either alone. Unfortunately, these combinations have been virtually withdrawn from the United States market. Often plain 1 per cent or 1.5 per cent hydrocortisone in ophthalmic ointment base suffices. If it doesn't, have the patient use the hydrocortisone topically in the morning and an antibiotic at bedtime, applying each one thinly. Tetracycline and erythromycin are safe for long-term topical use; avoid potentially sensitizing antibiotics such as neomycin.

CAUTION: **Glaucoma is a possible complication of topical corticosteroids used in the eyes.** The fluorinated corticosteroids seem to be more troublesome in this regard than hydrocortisone. Hydrocortisone ointment applied sparingly to the *eyelid edges only* with a clean fingertip has, in my experience, been safe in this regard. The patient should be instructed to apply a tiny amount to the eyelid edges with the eyes closed and keep it out of the eyes. Patients should also be told to interrupt their eyelid hydrocortisone application if they develop herpes simplex, because of the danger of developing herpetic keratitis.

Chest and back

A low- or medium-strength fluorinated corticosteroid cream, gel, or ointment—depending on the hairiness and dryness of the skin—applied spar-

Seborrheic dermatitis

ingly at bedtime or twice daily usually controls seborrheic dermatitis. Hydrocortisone tends to be relatively ineffective in this area. Be sure that the fluorinated corticosteroid is labeled "Do NOT use on face or skin-fold areas."

Armpits, groin, and breast folds

Seborrheic intertrigo (intertrigo is skin-fold dermatitis) is best treated with 1 per cent hydrocortisone cream. If candidiasis is present or suspected, the hydrocortisone can be compounded 1 per cent in a nystatin cream base. As an alternative, have the patient dust on nystatin powder very sparingly after thoroughly massaging in the hydrocortisone cream. Seborrheic intertrigo often responds poorly to 1 per cent hydrocortisone. If so, cautiously increase the hydrocortisone concentration to 2 per cent or even 3 per cent. Over a long period, this may cause slight thinning of the skin. Don't use fluorinated corticosteroids, because of their notorious tendency to cause skin thinning and striae when used in these skin folds. Such traditional antiseborrheic dermatitis remedies as tar and sulfur are poorly tolerated in the skin-fold areas of the armpits and groin; if you do try them, use them in a concentration of 1 per cent or less. These cautions apply to the skin-fold areas of the armpits and groin, but not to seborrheic dermatitis of the retroauricular fold. The areas behind the ears tolerate fluorinated corticosteroids and also topical sulfur, tars, and salicylic acid.

14

Dermatofibromas

Etiology

Dermatofibromas (histiocytomas) are firm, benign skin tumors whose cause is unknown. Left alone, dermatofibromas persist for decades. Some believe they represent a peculiar reaction to trauma, possibly insect bites. This theory offers a useful explanation for patients: "It's a scar reaction, probably from an old insect bite."

Diagnosis

The typical dermatofibroma is a smooth, hard, dome-shaped papule with a pink to violaceous to brownish color. These lesions occur in the dermis and give the epidermis a stretched appearance. They favor the extremities, especially the legs, and are more common in women than in men.

The history and appearance usually permit a clinical diagnosis. The principal differential diagnosis is that of a nevus, especially if lesions are enlarging or inflamed. As with any pigmented lesion, melanoma enters the differential diagnosis. Other malignancies, such as basal-cell carcinoma, squamous-cell carcinoma, or even fibrosarcoma, should be considered if the lesion is enlarging or atypical. It's sometimes impossible to distinguish a keloid or hypertrophic scar from a dermatofibroma.

Treatment

Reassurance is all that is needed unless you are unsure of the diagnosis or the patient is annoyed by the lesion. Dermatofibromas extend deep into the dermis; permanent removal requires full-thickness skin excision. Since these lesions are usually found on the extremities or trunk, the scar following excision is usually more prominent than the original dermatofibroma. If the diagnosis is in doubt, do a punch or shave biopsy. If you do a shave biopsy, be sure to explain to the patient that you are removing only the surface and the growth will probably recur.

Women often object to the protrusion of dermatofibromas, especially on the legs, where they interfere with shaving. Liquid nitrogen freezing is the best treatment for the protruding dermatofibroma. Moderately deep freezing is required since this is a dermal lesion. Explain to the patient that you are only flattening out the growth, and it may recur after some years. If so, it can be frozen again. The patient instruction sheet will help your patients live with dermatofibromas.

Dry skin (asteatosis, xerosis) | 15

Etiology

"Dry" skin is a common patient complaint. It occurs at all ages but becomes more of a problem with age. Many older patients chronically complain of dry, itchy skin. The legs are most commonly affected, but any body part may be.

Dry skin describes a clinical problem whose etiologic factors are incompletely understood. Skin moisture plays a central role; anything that causes the skin to lose moisture results in a tendency to dryness and chapping. The drier the air, the more rapidly skin moisture is lost. Consequently dry skin is a particular problem in cold winter climates where the warm indoor air is low in humidity. Removal of lipids and other skin components by soaps, detergents, and excessive bathing contributes to the damage. Dry skin begins with scaling and chapping; if it isn't checked, eczematous changes supervene and dominate the clinical picture. Frequently the patches of eczema are round and fairly sharply demarcated—the so-called nummular eczema. These round patches may be mistaken for ringworm. The patient may aggravate them by vigorous scrubbing or applying irritating remedies.

Diagnosis

Diagnosis is usually easy in the early stages, when there are mostly dryness, chapping, and low-grade erythema. Ichthyosis is the chief differential diagnosis. Ichthyosis is differentiated by its constant presence, its uniform morphology, and often a positive family history. When eczematous changes are present, it may be difficult to decide whether you're dealing with a primarily eczematous disorder associated with dry skin, or whether the eczematous changes are secondary to irritated dry skin. Dry skin is almost invariably present in atopic eczema and is a common accompaniment of psoriasis.

From the standpoint of treatment it makes little difference whether one is dealing with a primarily eczematous disorder with associated dry skin or with eczema superimposed on dry skin, since eczematous skin is treated similarly irrespective of the underlying problem. The prognosis, of course, is different: It's much more favorable if one is dealing simply with eczematous changes superimposed on dry skin.

Treatment

The treatment of dry skin must be in tune with its severity. Mild dryness and chapping respond well to skin hydration and lubricating measures. When dermatitis supervenes, topical corticosteroids should be added. When there is extensive, severe dermatitis, a three- to five-day tapering course of prednisone brings dramatic relief.

Skin hydration and lubrication

When there is only dryness and chapping, minimizing soap and simple measures to hydrate the skin are usually enough. Bath oils are an easy way to treat widespread dry skin. Bathing adds moisture to the skin; the oil film helps prevent loss of that moisture. Bath oils can be used in conjunction with showers; the oil is applied sparingly with the hands to the slightly moist, freshly dried skin after the shower. As bath oils produce a dangerously slippery tub, I prefer to have elderly patients apply the bath oil to their skin immediately after drying rather than add it to the bath water. There are many excellent bath oils on the market. A good approach is to give the patient several samples and suggest he purchase the one he likes best.

Patients with dry skin are frequently told to cut down on their baths; this isn't necessary unless they are bathing more than once daily. What is essential is that they not apply soap directly to their dry skin and that they lubricate their skin either immediately after their showers or baths or by adding bath oil to the bath water. Diluted soap running down the body with shower water is permissible.

Salad oil or hydrogenated vegetable cooking fats are sometimes recommended as inexpensive skin lubricants. They are safe and effective but often give clothes, pajamas, and towels an unpleasant, rancid odor. Mineral oil and plain petrolatum (Vaseline) don't do this. While mineral oil is a good, cheap substitute for bath oil applied to the skin, neither mineral nor vegetable oils are suitable for addition to bath water, since they lack the surfactant that makes the commercial bath oils miscible with water.

For mild, localized dry skin, many patients prefer lotions or creams. These provide moisture for skin hydration, and an oil to keep it there. Patient preferences vary widely. If you have samples, provide them for patient trial. Otherwise write down a number of lubricants that seem to be favorites among your patients; avoid the more widely advertised ones. Some "dry skin" preparations contain urea or lactic acid. These additives supposedly help the skin retain moisture and increase its smoothness. However, prolonged use may cause irritation.

Corticosteroid therapy

When eczematous changes are present, a topical corticosteroid should be applied sparingly four to five times a day. Ointments are usually more effective than creams or lotions. If an ointment is applied sparingly and massaged in well, it isn't too messy. For fastidious patients, a useful compromise is to prescribe a cream or lotion for use during the day and a greasy corticosteroid at bedtime. If you don't wish to burden the patient with the expense of purchasing two medications, have him apply plain petrolatum at bedtime after thoroughly massaging in the corticosteroid cream.

Systemic treatment is needed only in rare, severe cases of dry-skin dermatitis. Here a brief, two- to five-day tapering course of prednisone brings dramatic relief and is more practical than whole-body application of topical corticosteroids. Start with 40 to 60 mg of prednisone taken in one dose on the first day, and then decrease it by 10 to 20 mg a day over the next two to four days. Antihistamines and other so-called antipruritics are of no value. At best, they sedate the patient so the itching is less worrisome. It's preferable to treat the cause.

Managing the patient

Success in managing dry-skin dermatitis requires compliance and the patient's understanding that lubricating measures may be required for a long time. The patient instruction sheet will help get this message across. Stress that dry-skin dermatitis tends to recur and that the patient should resume the hydrating and lubricating measures at the first sign of dry skin.

16

5-Fluorouracil

5-Fluorouracil (5-FU) is a cytotoxic agent with selective toxicity for sun-damaged cells. This selective action is the basis for its clinical usefulness: It can destroy sun-damaged skin with little injury to normal tissue. Healing takes place by replication of the remaining epidermal and adnexal cells; effective 5-FU treatment requires significant skin destruction.

Skin destruction leads to the major complication of 5-FU treatment—patient noncompliance. Patients intensely dislike this treatment, since for two to three weeks the treated area is raw and unsightly. There is often considerable discomfort. Properly selected patients will be delighted with the final result, although they sometimes complain bitterly during treatment. Complaints can be minimized by explaining the need for skin destruction and by showing photographs of patients undergoing treatment. The patient instruction sheet helps.

A second drawback to topical 5-FU therapy is the absence of a definite treatment endpoint. Treatment is stopped when the physician estimates that sufficient destruction has occurred. Estimates of the time required for adequate 5-FU treatment are provided in the unit on actinic keratoses; however, the length of treatment must be tailored to the individual patient.

Detailed instructions for the use of 5-FU are also given in the unit on actinic keratoses. The following points are worth remembering:

1. Topical 5-FU destroys actinic keratoses but has no effect on seborrheic keratoses or warts.
2. Lesions that respond only partially or not at all to one course of 5-FU should not be retreated with 5-FU. Biopsy is mandatory to rule out carcinoma.
3. Topical 5-FU is not adequate treatment for skin cancer. Even superficial basal-cell carcinoma should not be treated with commercial 5-FU.
4. Topical 5-FU, while effective on the face, requires modification for actinic keratoses in other locations, such as the hands and forearms.

Fragile skin bleeding

17

Etiology

Senile purpura is the standard term for the tendency to ecchymoses and purpura of the dorsa of hands and forearms that annoys many older persons. Substitute the phrase *fragile skin bleeding* for the pejorative *senile purpura,* since it isn't a result of senility but comes from solar damage to the connective tissue of the skin. As a result of the degenerative changes in the connective tissue, even trivial shearing may cause an extensive ecchymosis.

Diagnosis

The diagnosis is obvious at a glance, since the bleeding is limited to the dorsa of the hands and forearms and spares the volar aspects of the forearms and the remaining skin. Purpura and ecchymoses secondary to connective-tissue damage sometimes occur in systemic disorders such as rheumatoid arthritis and may also be seen as a result of prolonged corticosteroid administration. Differentiate such conditions by examining the legs, since the purpura of rheumatoid arthritis and corticosteroid damage affects the legs while the purpura of solar damage spares them.

Treatment

This condition is permanent; there is no effective treatment. Do reassure patients that the condition is the result of localized skin damage and not a sign of a blood disorder or other serious illness. It usually suffices to tell patients that the bleeding is a result of sun damage to the skin and ask them to read the information sheet for further details. The patient information sheet encourages patients to minimize future sun damage; also give them the sheet titled "Sunlight and Your Skin."

18

Herpes simplex

Etiology

Herpes simplex infections are caused by the herpes hominis virus, which has two distinct strains, HSV 1 and HSV 2. Genital herpes is usually caused by type 2 virus, while the type 1 strain is responsible for most facial infections.

The initial infection with herpesvirus, or primary herpes simplex infection, generally produces a painful, marked local reaction along with such systemic symptoms as fever and malaise. Type 1 primary herpes simplex infection usually occurs in children as an inflammation of the oral mucosa and gums. It sometimes occurs in adults as well. The typical grouped blisters of herpes may not be evident in primary herpetic gingivostomatitis, and new, isolated vesicles can continue to erupt for days. The primary attack of genital herpes is painful and associated with systemic symptoms, especially in women, in whom it may produce severe vulvovaginitis. Primary genital herpes is mostly a disease seen in adults, since it's usually acquired through sexual intercourse.

Following the primary infection, the virus establishes residence in a nerve root ganglion and may periodically travel down the nerve to the skin to produce recurrent disease. These recurring groups of blisters, herpes simplex recurrens, are the most common clinical presentation of herpes simplex.

Diagnosis

Primary herpes simplex is often misdiagnosed as "infection" (Figures C-19 and C-20), cellulitis, insect bite, or even contact dermatitis. Herpes simplex recurrens is usually readily diagnosed; crops of blisters on an erythematous base appear in a similar area with each attack. Most patients with recurrent herpes appear with their own correct diagnosis and want treatment. In the early stages, before significant blistering occurs, and in the later phases, when only erosions or crusts may be present, diagnosis can be difficult and herpes may perfectly resemble a nonspecific dermatitis or a pyoderma. Extensive herpes simplex recurrens may resemble herpes zoster or an acute

93

vesicular contact dermatitis. Herpes simplex presenting in more unusual locations, such as the fingers, may be misdiagnosed because of failure to consider that possibility.

Herpes simplex recurrens of the genitalia is often atypical in its appearance and may present diagnostic difficulties. The clinically diagnosable stage of grouped vesicles may be transient or may not appear at all. Any recurring erosions, rash, or sores in the genital area should be suspected of being herpes simplex.

Herpes simplex is essentially a clinical diagnosis. The virus can be cultured from active lesions, and this specialized procedure is available in most urban areas. The cells at the bases of the vesicles of herpes simplex, herpes zoster, and varicella show alterations in morphology. Cellular material can be obtained by unroofing a blister and gently scraping the base with a clean blade after soaking up the blister fluid with sterile gauze. The cellular debris is smeared thinly on a slide and stained with Giemsa or Wright's stain.

Herpes simplex, herpes zoster, and varicella produce identical changes, consisting of huge, multinucleated giant cells many times the size of an epidermal cell, as well as nuclear inclusion bodies. When present, the virally caused giant cells are obvious.

Complications

Primary herpes simplex infection of neonates and young infants is serious and may be fatal. In patients with eczematous disorders both primary and recurrent herpes may become generalized, a disorder called eczema herpeticum. Some of these patients become very ill. Patients on immunosuppressants may develop progressive, atypical herpes infections.

Ophthalmic herpes simplex is justifiably dreaded since it may cause corneal ulcerations that can progress to scarring and blindness. Topical corticosteroids aggravate herpetic eye disease and are contraindicated in ophthalmic herpes. A deleterious effect of topical corticosteroids has been documented only for ophthalmic herpes. No clear-cut effect—either beneficial or adverse—has been shown for corticosteroids applied to cutaneous herpes.

An occasional complication of recurrent herpes simplex is erythema multiforme. This hypersensitivity reaction usually appears a few days after the onset of the herpes. It may be severe enough to overshadow the herpetic infection completely. It responds dramatically to systemic corticosteroids.

The yellow crusting stage of herpes simplex is sometimes mistaken for a bacterial infection and treated with topical or systemic antibiotics. Bacterial superinfection of herpes appears to be rare; usually petrolatum lubrication during the crusting stage is all that's needed.

Contagion

Herpes infections are contagious to those who haven't previously been infected. Few individuals escape type 1 infection during childhood. Contagion of type 1 herpes is uncommon among adults. Not so with the "genital" type 2 virus, which is epidemic among sexually active adults. The traditional advice that this is contagious only when lesions are present may be incorrect; both men and women may shed virus when free of visible lesions. Whether the virus can be transmitted during symptom-free stages is not known.

Treatment

There is no present effective prophylactic treatment for cutaneous herpes simplex, either type 1 or type 2. For ocular herpes topical antiviral agents (idoxuridine, vidarabine) are of definite benefit. The innumerable therapeutic attempts at dealing with herpes have used two approaches: (1) measures to alter the body's immune status and (2) topical applications to the lesions, aimed at destroying or inactivating the virus. Patients with herpes simplex recurrens already have high titers of circulating antivirus antibodies; vaccinations aimed at producing antibodies have no effect.

As evidence of our therapeutic impotence, new therapies for herpes simplex have appeared frequently, only to join the long list of discarded remedies when their lack of value finally becomes evident. Acyclovir (Zovirax), a new antiviral drug, is *not* effective for recurrent herpes, although it may shorten the course of primary herpes simplex. This expensive drug should not be used in recurrent attacks of herpes, as resistant strains have already appeared.

Herpes simplex recurrens may be variable, with one attack succeeding another for months, and then—without apparent reason—the victim is spared further episodes for a year or more. Equally unpredictable is the severity of individual attacks. An episode of herpes may be mild, with a few small evanescent blisters that disappear within days, or it may be severe and involve much of the lips, with huge blisters and crusts that leave the patient miserable for more than two weeks.

A rare complication of herpes simplex is erythema multiforme. In predisposed individuals, this hypersensitivity reaction may follow each attack of herpes simplex recurrens. The erythema multiforme caused by herpes simplex may be severe, with widespread blistering. Fortunately, it responds to adequate doses of systemic corticosteroids.

Complications of treatment

Complications of treatment are invariably the result of inappropriate treatment. Irritant dermatitis from over-the-counter remedies is fairly common. Allergic dermatitis from a topical antibiotic applied to treat supposed secondary infection occurs occasionally. Because of the risk of herpetic keratitis, topical corticosteroids should never be used on herpes of the eye.

Managing the patient

What can you offer the patient? Reassure him that herpes does not scar. During the acute vesicular stage bland compresses will soothe; directions for dilute vinegar compresses are given in the patient instruction sheet. Dryness and painful fissuring when crusts have formed are relieved by sparing applications of petrolatum. Discourage the use of the many over-the-counter cold-sore remedies. Many are irritating, some can actually cause allergic dermatitis, and all are worthless.

Herpes of the lips and face is often triggered by sunlight. Suitable sun protectives—described in the patient information sheet "Sunlight and Your Skin"—often benefit patients whose herpes appears after a skiing trip or a beach outing.

Recurrent herpes of the genitalia is particularly trying; often the friction of sexual intercourse triggers another attack. Abstinence is hardly a satisfactory solution. Use of lubricants during intercourse sometimes helps. Explain to patients that attacks of genital herpes may eventually become less frequent and finally cease.

Herpes simplex

Herpes zoster (shingles)

19

Etiology

Herpes zoster results from the activation of varicella (chickenpox) virus dormant in the body. The mechanism of activation is unknown; the majority of patients with herpes zoster are otherwise healthy. While textbooks stress the association of shingles with lymphomas, other neoplastic disease, and immunosuppressants, a thorough search for systemic disease in healthy-appearing persons with herpes zoster is not warranted.

When herpes zoster is accompanied by widespread disseminated lesions, a search for underlying disease is indicated. Widespread dissemination—in other words, an accompanying varicella—is often the consequence of damage to the patient's immune system. A few disseminated lesions may be disregarded, as it isn't uncommon to see a few vesicles at a distance from the neural distribution of herpes zoster.

Diagnosis

Only a glance is required for diagnosis of the linear patches of grouped vesicles on an erythematous base, stopping sharply at the midline. Difficulties may be encountered in the early stages of herpes zoster, before blistering has become evident, when the red, infiltrated, sharply demarcated, sometimes painful patches may suggest bacterial cellulitis, an insect-bite reaction, or even a fixed drug eruption. The appearance of blisters in the next day or two usually corrects the diagnosis. Herpes zoster in the blistering stage is occasionally misdiagnosed as a severe contact dermatitis. Linear herpes simplex may closely resemble herpes zoster, but the presence of intense burning or pain favors the diagnosis of the latter.

The neuralgia of shingles may precede the skin eruption by a week or more. Patients may complain of a painful "strained back" preceding their herpes zoster of the trunk. Sometimes the history of marked burning or pain in the affected area *before* the rash breaks out is useful in the differential diagnosis of early herpes zoster. While recurrent herpes simplex is sometimes preceded by tingling or itching in the affected area, usually it's mild and is present less than a day before the rash appears.

Contagion

Patients with herpes zoster should be considered as contagious as if they had varicella. They are potentially contagious to infants and small children who have never had varicella, as well as to any adult whose immune system has been altered by illness and/or drugs. In particular, patients must scrupulously avoid anyone with malignancies or on long-term corticosteroids or immunosuppressants (kidney transplant, systemic LE, and the like).

Treatment

In the absence of a specific anti-varicella-virus drug, treatment remains symptomatic. Dilute acetic acid (white vinegar) compresses are a simple, inexpensive treatment for blisters and crusts. The technique is described in the patient instruction sheet. Dryness and fissuring during the later healing stages are relieved by sparing applications of white petrolatum (Vaseline).

The neuralgia of herpes zoster is the real therapeutic challenge. The pain may be excruciating and may continue after the skin eruption has healed. The neuralgia of shingles tends to be more severe in older persons. In younger patients the neuralgia is usually mild and transient.

Treatment of the neuralgia requires adequate analgesics. I usually use aspirin or acetaminophen (Tylenol) for mild pain. For moderate pain, I combine 30 to 60 mg of codeine with these agents. Very severe pain requires oral meperidine (Demerol). In most patients, severe pain is short-lived, and I use narcotic analgesics if they're necessary to provide relief.

Systemic corticosteroids effectively shorten the course of severe herpes zoster neuralgia and appear to lessen the possibility of postherpetic neuralgia. Many remedies have been advocated for these purposes, but only systemic corticosteroids have been proven effective by well-controlled studies. I use systemic corticosteroids in older persons with significant neuralgia unless there's a significant contraindication, such as an active peptic ulcer or bacterial infection. A common regimen is three weeks of prednisone: 60 mg daily the first week, 40 mg daily the second week, and 20 mg daily the third week. The daily prednisone should be taken as one dose in the morning. Some flexibility is wise; the course can be shortened if the neuralgia clears promptly, while stubborn cases may benefit from one to three weeks longer on the steroid. There appears to be little benefit from continuing systemic corticosteroids for more than six weeks.

In addition to adequate analgesics and systemic prednisone, patients often benefit from a mild sedative at bedtime. Barbiturates are best avoided; preferred drugs are promethazine (Phenergan), hydroxyzine (Vistaril, Atarax), chlordiazepoxide (Librium), diazepam (Valium), or similar mild, nonbarbiturate sedating agents.

What about the minority of patients whose neuralgia is not controlled with analgesics, systemic corticosteroids, and possibly mild sedatives? Most of the recommended measures fail, with one pleasant exception: Chlorprothixene, a psychotherapeutic agent related to the phenothiazines, has worked in a number of my patients who had previously tried everything. The original study on this agent[1] reported the drug to be extremely effective in herpes zoster neuralgia, and subsequent reports have confirmed its value.[2,3] The doses originally recommended were 50 mg by mouth every six hours for moderate pain and 100 mg four times daily for severe neuralgia. Because of its phenothiazine-like action, I've found it preferable to initiate dosage at somewhat lower levels—25 mg four times daily—and increase it if improvement isn't evident in a few days. Drowsiness and other side effects are prominent with chlorprothixene; acquaint yourself with the side effects listed in the product-information brochure. Because of possible severe sedation, it may be desirable to initiate chlorprothixene therapy in the hospital. While in the original study on chlorprothixene the drug was apparently used for 10 days or less, some of my patients have required it for longer periods.

Complications

Herpes zoster sometimes leaves scars. On the skin, scars are usually mild and only a modest cosmetic handicap; in the eyes they can prove disastrous. Ophthalmic herpes zoster is a serious emergency requiring ophthalmologic consultation. Zoster of the eyelid doesn't necessarily mean that the eye is involved. If, however, the patient reports pain in the eye itself, or if the bulbar conjunctiva is inflamed, ophthalmologic consultation is imperative. Sometimes severe swelling of the eyelid makes it difficult to evaluate the condition of the eye; when this happens, I prefer to play it safe and have an ophthalmologic colleague see the patient.

While herpes zoster is usually limited to the sensory nerves, motor nerves may be involved, with disturbances of urination, muscle weakness, or paralysis. This is usually localized and limited and clears spontaneously.

Postherpetic neuralgia is often a distressing and lengthy complication—it can go on for years. If the patient hasn't had a course of systemic corticosteroids, they should be tried. Chlorprothixene is often effective. Nerve blocks and even neurosurgical procedures have been recommended; I've had no experience with them. Sometimes reassurance and analgesics are all you can offer. Because postherpetic neuralgia is often a long-term problem, bear in mind the habituating effects of potent analgesics and strong sedatives.

References

1. Farber GA, Burks JW: Chlorprothixene therapy for herpes zoster neuralgia. *South Med J* 67:808, 1974

2. Nathan PW: Chlorprothixene (Taractan) in post-herpetic neuralgia and other severe chronic pains. *Pain* 5:367, 1978

3. Kramer PW: The management of postherpetic neuralgia with chlorprothixene. *Surg Neurol* 15:102, 1981

20

Hives (urticaria)

Etiology

Acute urticaria is a common problem and usually responds dramatically to medications. The patient information sheet is designed for those with acute urticaria. Chronic urticaria is an infinitely more complex problem that can't be covered in a routine patient information sheet. This discussion is limited to acute urticaria. Those wishing to improve their ability to struggle with chronic urticaria will benefit from reading the monograph by Warin and Champion[1] as well as a more recent review.[2]

Urticaria is a nonspecific vascular reaction of the skin. Patients and physicians tend to equate hives with allergy. However, many cases of urticaria have a pharmacologic basis, as certain foods (strawberries) or drugs (codeine) have an innate urticariogenic action. Cholinergic urticaria, with its small papules triggered by heat or physical or emotional stress, is an endogenous pharmacologic phenomenon. Exogenous physical factors such as cold, heat, pressure, or light can all cause urticaria.

Urticaria may be related to an underlying disease such as infections, collagen diseases, or neoplasia. If a patient with acute urticaria reports malaise or systemic symptoms, an underlying infectious process must be ruled out. Urticaria itches but usually doesn't cause other significant symptoms.

Diagnosis

Urticaria is defined as transient wheals; the transient nature of the lesion is an important part of the definition. Individual hives usually develop and recede within a few hours. Often the diagnosis is made from the history, as hives may be absent at the time of examination. When hivelike lesions persist for more than a few hours, the eruption is not true urticaria.

From the standpoint of therapy, it's important to limit the diagnosis of urticaria to lesions lasting only hours. True urticaria usually responds to antihistamines and epinephrine. The fixed erythemas, such as erythema multiforme, are usually unaffected by antihistamines and require corticosteroids for suppression. Not infrequently patients report wheals that persist for 12 hours or more and show a clinical picture intermediate between true urticaria and the classical fixed erythemas. Such intermediate forms have been termed erythema-group reactions; they resemble fixed erythemas in responding to systemic corticosteroids but not to antihistamines.

Treatment

Assuming that you've asked the patient to stop any suspected drugs or foods and have ruled out an underlying infectious process, treatment boils down to suppressing the eruption with drugs. Stopping "any suspected drug" is easier said than done when you encounter patients who are taking numerous drugs for serious illnesses. In this situation, eliminate all nonessential drugs (e.g., barbiturates, aspirin), treat the patient with urticaria suppressants, and hope for the best.

Patients with urticaria should not take aspirin or aspirin-containing medicines. Allergy to aspirin may cause hives. Even in those not allergic to it, aspirin tends to aggravate hives pharmacologically.

Antihistamines are the best drugs for suppressing urticaria. Antihistamines can be divided into chemical groups; when two antihistamines are employed, they should be from different chemical classes. Widely used groups are the alkylamines (chlorpheniramine, Chlor-Trimeton; brompheniramine, Dimetane; triprolidine, Actidil), ethanolamines (diphenhydramine, Benadryl), hydroxyzine (Atarax, Vistaril), and phenothiazine (promethazine, Phenergan; cyproheptadine, Periactin). It's neither necessary nor desirable to employ many different antihistamines. Limit yourself to one or two antihistamines from each of these groups, and become familiar with them.

Keep two things in mind in prescribing antihistamines: (1) Patients with urticaria may require two to three times the "usual" adult dose, and (2) antihistamines vary in their central-nervous-system side effects. The more sedating antihistamines such as diphenhydramine, hydroxyzine, promethazine, and cyproheptadine are preferably used at bedtime.

For daytime I prefer either chlorpheniramine or brompheniramine in a dose of 8 mg (two *regular* tablets) three times daily at mealtime (for convenience). The patient is told to decrease the dosage to one tablet three times daily if he gets too sleepy and to increase it to three tablets three times daily if the hives are only partially suppressed. Do not use long-acting tablet forms for daytime treatment of acute urticaria. Their delayed onset and cumulative effect make dosage adjustment difficult.

At bedtime I frequently have the patient take a more sedating and/or longer-acting antihistamine and prefer 25 or 50 mg of hydroxyzine. Promethazine, 12.5 or 25 mg at bedtime, is also very useful. If the urticaria is mild, the daytime antihistamine given additionally at bedtime usually suffices. The long-acting tablets of chlorpheniramine or brompheniramine can be used at bedtime to keep the patient comfortable overnight.

CAUTION: **Antihistamines may cause drowsiness;** warn patients that it may be dangerous to drive or perform similar tasks requiring alertness and tell them not to consume alcohol while taking antihistamines. Antihistamines may cause urinary retention in older men; try smaller doses first.

Once control of hives is achieved, the patient should continue the same dose for an additional two or three days before gradually decreasing the antihistamines. This schedule is arbitrary and needs to be individualized, but generally it's wise to allow a 7- to 12-day period of gradually decreasing the antihistamine dose before stopping. Any urticarial flare-up while tapering the antihistamine requires an increase in dosage.

Epinephrine, 0.3 ml of a 1:1,000 dilution injected subcutaneously or intramuscularly, is an effective immediate treatment for severe acute urticaria. It's preferable to avoid epinephrine in patients with hypertension or cardiac disease. A beneficial effect is usually evident in 30 to 40 minutes. Patients responding well to epinephrine usually do well on antihistamines. Those failing to respond to epinephrine will usually require corticosteroids to control their wheals.

Other sympathomimetic drugs, such as ephedrine or pseudoephedrine (Sudafed), may be given by mouth. For severe urticaria I generally use them in addition to antihistamines. As these agents often cause jitteriness, they are best taken only at breakfast and lunch. The dose of ephedrine is 25 to 50 mg, and for pseudoephedrine, 30 to 60 mg.

Corticosteroids are occasionally necessary to suppress hives. In general, urticaria responds better to antihistamines than to corticosteroids. Some cases don't do well with antihistamines but clear up promptly with corticosteroids. If wheals last more than a few hours, if joint swelling accompanies urticaria (serum sickness syndrome), or if there's no response to epinephrine, systemic corticosteroids will usually be required.

Prednisone is the corticosteroid of choice and, as it's relatively short-acting, may initially be required twice daily before the patient switches to the usual once-daily morning dose. Start with enough corticosteroid to suppress the hives; usually between 60 and 100 mg of prednisone are required initially. Once control is achieved, taper the dose by 5 to 10 mg a day over a 10- to 12-day period.

Corticosteroids should be used reluctantly, and only if antihistamines fail. Not only may corticosteroids mask an underlying disease process, but they interfere with the body's anti-infection mechanisms. Before using corticosteroids, rule out an infectious process; a blood count, urinalysis, and sedimentation rate are minimum laboratory tests. If more than two weeks of corticosteroids are required, a thorough medical reassessment is indicated.

References

1. Warin RP, Champion RH: *Urticaria*. Philadelphia: Saunders, 1974
2. Monroe EW, Jones HE: Urticaria: An updated review. *Arch Dermatol* 113:80, 1977

21

Impetigo

Etiology

Impetigo is a superficial cutaneous coccal infection. The relative roles of streptococci and staphylococci remain controversial and are mostly of academic interest. Impetigo virtually always responds to erythromycin or penicillin—even when antibiotic-resistant staphylococci are cultured from it.

Impetigo can occur at any age; in North America it's predominantly a disorder of children. It's customary to inquire as to staphylococcal or streptococcal infections (impetigo, furuncles, strep throat) among family members and playmates in an attempt to discover a source of infection. Such sources should be examined and treated; usually no contagious source is found.

Diagnosis

Diagnosis of typical cases of impetigo is easy. The enlarging lesions with actively blistering or crusted borders and central clearing (Figure C-21) resemble few other disorders. Inflammatory tinea corporis (ringworm) caused by zoophilic fungi contracted from a pet or farm animal can produce a clinical picture morphologically resembling impetigo. Usually tinea develops more slowly than impetigo. In bullous impetigo, blisters persist (instead of rupturing early and leaving crusts) and other vesicular disorders have to be considered. Herpes simplex, herpes zoster, varicella, and severe blistering contact dermatitis are occasionally mistaken for impetigo.

Impetigo is by definition a superficial bacterial infection of the skin. Deeper pyodermas, termed ecthyma, are not impetigo. Considerable confusion has arisen as to treatment and complications of impetigo because some studies have failed to make this distinction.

Contagion

Impetigo contagiosa—the full name of this disorder—is indeed contagious. Therefore, children with this disorder should be kept home from school for two days after the start of treatment. Parents should be advised as to contagiousness, and simple hygienic measures instituted as outlined in the patient instruction sheet. Usually the crusting, contagious stage of impetigo clears up with two days of systemic antibiotics.

Complications

Streptococcal skin infections, like streptococcal infections elsewhere, may result in glomerulonephritis. The incidence of glomerulonephritis depends not only on the presence of nephritogenic strains of streptococci, but on how long the pyoderma had been present before treatment. Nephritis as a complication of impetigo is rare in North American private practice. Reports showing relatively high incidences of glomerulonephritis have usually dealt with children raised in poverty-stricken surroundings with neglected lesions. Often what is reported as "impetigo" actually represents long-standing deep pyodermas. I see no point in needlessly alarming patients and parents by mentioning the possibility of kidney disease.

Treatment

Impetigo is a delight to treat; the response to systemic antibiotics is dramatic. A five- to seven-day course of erythromycin or penicillin by mouth generally suffices. There seems no need to subject the patient to the discomfort of intramuscular penicillin with its increased risk of adverse reactions.

The effectiveness of topical antibiotics remains controversial. Many physicians believe that the average case of impetigo requires only topical antibiotics. There are studies stating that topical antibiotics are without effect in impetigo; however, it appears that these workers were treating deeper pyodermas and not impetigo, which is a very superficial process. The bulk of evidence indicates that topical antibiotics are effective in true impetigo.

Which are more effective, systemic or topical antibiotics? There's no doubt: Systemic antibiotics are invariably more effective. I prefer to use both systemic and topical antibiotics. Why add a topical antibiotic when systemic antibiotics are so effective? This personal preference is not irrational; patients don't always take their systemic antibiotics as directed. Furthermore, many patients want something to put on their skin. If you fail to prescribe or advise a specific product, they're likely to apply some irritating material.

Systemic therapy

A wide variety of antibiotics are effective in treating impetigo. I prefer erythromycin or a semisynthetic, orally effective penicillin such as cloxacillin or dicloxacillin. A five-day course of antibiotic usually suffices; I make the prescription refillable once and tell the patient that if the impetigo doesn't completely clear, he should have the prescription refilled and take a second five-day course. Emphasize the importance of taking the entire five-day supply of antibiotic and not stopping in a day or two, when the lesions are better.

Impetigo

Topical therapy

Gentle removal of crusts is important. While lukewarm water works well for this purpose, patients are more likely to comply if something is added to the water. Dilute acetic acid in the form of white vinegar fulfills the need for a harmless, cheap additive. The patient information sheet gives instructions for preparing the vinegar-water mixture. Soaking is stopped once crusts no longer form.

A nonsensitizing antibiotic ointment should be applied thinly three to four times a day until healing is complete. When there are crusts, the ointment should be applied after the crusts have been soaked off. I generally use a bacitracin-polymyxin combination (Polysporin) or oxytetracycline (Terramycin) ointment. Neomycin is best avoided, as it sensitizes, and such antibiotics as gentamicin (Garamycin) are best reserved for systemic treatment of severe infections.

Impetigo clears up in one week. Patients should be told to return if not fine by then. Failure to clear in a week can usually be traced to (1) failure to take the antibiotic, (2) a wrong diagnosis, or (3) superimposition of the impetigo on another process, such as contact dermatitis, which is still present.

22

Keloids

Etiology

Keloids are tumors of excessive scar tissue. Obvious skin injury—surgery, an accidental cut, an insect bite, a pimple—usually precedes keloid formation. Occasionally the initiating injury is so trivial it escapes notice; these are "spontaneous" keloids. Keloids are more likely to occur in dark-skinned persons and in certain areas of the body, especially the upper chest and upper back. For additional details, a recent review[1] is highly recommended.

Diagnosis

The smooth, sharply circumscribed, elevated tumor is usually diagnostic, especially if there are multiple lesions. A history of preceding trauma supports the diagnosis. Sometimes tumors, either benign (e.g., dermatofibroma) or malignant (e.g., infiltrating basal-cell carcinoma), may resemble keloids. If in doubt, do a small punch biopsy. Distinction between hypertrophic scars and keloids, put forward by some texts, is probably not realistic since there is no demarcation between hypertrophic scars and keloids.

Treatment

Patients seek treatment of keloids because of their appearance or discomfort. Keloids, especially those on the trunk, may cause significant, persistent burning, discomfort, or pain. Textbooks correctly describe the treatment of keloids as unsatisfactory. It's easier to list what not to do. Surgery is best avoided; a new and larger keloid is often the result.

Intralesional repository corticosteroids constitute the best present-day treatment. They usually are promptly effective in eliminating keloidal pain and discomfort, but flatten out the keloid only slowly. Multiple treatments are usually necessary. Explain to the patient that the injections will not eliminate the keloid, but will make it flatter and less noticeable. Even successful treatment leaves a flat, shiny scar.

Local anesthesia before the intralesional injection is recommended unless the keloid is tiny. Triamcinolone acetonide suspension is the repository corticosteroid most widely used. Start with the 10 mg/ml concentration (Kenalog-10). The corticosteroid should be injected fairly deeply (5 to 8 mm) into the keloid. This requires considerable pressure on the plunger of the tuberculin syringe, which should be equipped with a Luer-Lok device to prevent separation of the needle from the syringe. Inject 0.1 to 0.2 ml of suspension at 5- to 10-mm intervals along the keloid. Limit the amount of triamcinolone acetonide injected to less than 20 to 30 mg.

The patient should be re-evaluated in two months. The repository corticosteroid acts for about three months, and works slowly. At the follow-up visit, injections can be repeated, using the 40 mg/ml concentration (Kenalog-40) if there was no response to 10 mg/ml. CAUTION: **The 40 mg/ml concentration increases the risk of skin atrophy.** Inject no more than 0.1 ml of this at a site, and at least 5 mm deep. With careful, repeated intralesional corticosteroid injections, most keloids cease causing discomfort and *gradually* flatten out. Sometimes, months or years after a keloid has successfully yielded to intralesional corticosteroids, it recurs. Inject it again.

Intralesional corticosteroids may cause undesirable local and systemic side effects. The injected drug is absorbed; large amounts may cause significant adrenal suppression. Cutaneous atrophy, depigmentation, telangiectasis, and even ulceration may occur as a result of the atrophy-promoting effects of corticosteroids. Local side effects are more likely with higher concentrations and if the drug is injected intradermally. Intralesional corticosteroids should be injected *sub*dermally at a depth of 5 to 8 mm.

Other treatments for keloids include radiation, pressure, topical retinoic acid, and freezing with liquid nitrogen or Dry Ice. None is as simple and effective as intralesional corticosteroids. Some workers combine a destructive method, such as liquid nitrogen freezing, with intralesional corticosteroids. There is no documented benefit of this dual approach.

Prevention

Is it possible to prevent postoperative keloids in those prone to form them? Radiation, while effective, requires a significant dose, about 1,500 to 2,000 rad. Most physicians, and patients, are opposed to radiation for benign conditions. Intralesional corticosteroids may prevent postoperative keloids. At surgery, a fairly dilute (5 to 10 mg/ml) suspension of triamcinolone acetonide is injected into the wound edges. Further steroid is usually injected two to four weeks postoperatively. Because corticosteroids inhibit wound healing, caution is necessary.

Reference

1. Murray JC, Pollack S, Pinell SR: Keloids: A review. *J Am Acad Dermatol* 4:461, 1981

Patient sheets pages P-51, P-59, P-61, P-67

Molluscum contagiosum 23

Etiology

Molluscum contagiosum is characterized by small skin tumors caused by a poxvirus. While more common in the young, it may affect persons of any age. Molluscum contagiosum is becoming an increasingly common sexually transmitted disease affecting the genitalia, abdomen, thighs, and buttocks.

Diagnosis

Molluscum lesions (Figure C-22) are shiny, white to flesh-colored, dome-shaped lesions with a firm, waxy appearance. When well developed, they have a diagnostic central indentation or umbilication. The tiny, early lesions often lack this feature. Most molluscum lesions are smaller than 5 mm, although occasional lesions are larger.

Molluscum lesions may undergo spontaneous inflammation, which may be mistaken for a bacterial infection. At times a low-grade rash surrounds molluscum lesions; with removal of the lesions, the rash clears.

Molluscum lesions are most commonly misdiagnosed as warts. Unlike warts, however, they are smooth, and careful observation with low-power magnification will reveal the diagnostic central pit. It's easy to misdiagnose a solitary molluscum lesion, especially when it's inflamed. Pyogenic granuloma, inflamed cyst, keratoacanthoma, inflamed wart, and basal-cell carcinoma are errors I have made. Superficial biopsy suffices, since histology reveals the characteristic molluscum bodies within the lesion.

Treatment

Locally destructive measures are the only effective treatment since we lack a systemic anti-molluscum-virus agent. Fortunately, molluscum lesions respond nicely to a variety of destructive therapies. They are easier to treat than warts.

Application of the blistering agent cantharidin is a gentle, painless treatment, and my first choice. Cantharidin is commercially available dissolved in flexible collodion under the trade name Cantharone. A minute drop is applied to each lesion with a pointed stick; a toothpick is ideal. Allow at least five minutes for thorough drying and caution the patient to expect a blister or irritation at each site. Have the patient return in 10 to 14 days, at which time most of the molluscum lesions will have disappeared. Repeat the cantharidin painting. Usually two to four treatments suffice. CAUTION: **The genitals are sensitive to this blistering agent.** Use minute amounts of cantharidin in treating the genitalia, and be certain that the patient remains still for five minutes to ensure drying. The same caution applies to small children. In some, cantharidin works poorly. Its effect can be potentiated by covering treated sites *after drying* with an occlusive tape such as Blenderm tape.

If you don't have cantharidin on hand, almost any superficial destructive measure will work. The lesions can be lightly curetted or superficially snipped off with a sharp scissors. They can be slit open with a small, sterile hypodermic needle and the contents squeezed out with a comedo extractor or a forceps. Liquid nitrogen freezing can be used. However, the various proprietary irritant wart topicals often fail in treating molluscum lesions.

Molluscum lesions tend to disappear spontaneously. In an occasional patient, such as an uncooperative small child with lesions on the eyelids, it's best to explain this tendency toward natural cure, and do nothing.

24

Nevi

Etiology

The word nevus is used in two ways. *Nevus* in a general sense refers to any circumscribed, persistent, genetically determined skin malformation. More often, it is used in a restricted way to describe a tumor or aggregation of melanocytes (nevus cells). The lay term "mole" usually corresponds to nevus-cell tumors. Other forms of nevi—hemangiomas, organoid nevi, connective-tissue nevi—are usually referred to as "birthmarks" in lay terminology. The congenital melanocytic nevus, being present at birth, is usually included in the birthmark category rather than called a mole.

The number and location of melanocytic nevi are genetically determined. "Moley" parents tend to have "moley" children. The common nevus is rare at birth. It appears as a flat brown spot during infancy or childhood and gradually becomes more prominent. Often melanocytic nevi appear in crops, or showers, especially in late childhood and during adolescence.

The congenital melanocytic nevus, although composed of melanocytes, differs from the usual melanocytic nevus. Congenital nevi, present at birth, enlarge in proportion to the growth of the infant and child. Unlike the usual nevi, congenital nevi have a significant potential for transformation into malignant melanomas (Figure C-27). The larger the congenital nevus, the greater the risk of transformation into a malignant melanoma. While everyone agrees that giant congenital nevi have a significant incidence of malignant transformation, we are unsure how often smaller congenital nevi become malignant.

Pathologically, nevi are classified by the location of the melanocytes. A nevus with melanocytes found at the dermo-epidermal junction is called a junctional nevus. Melanocytes restricted to the dermis form a dermal nevus. A nevus formed of both junctional and dermal cells is a compound nevus. When nevus cells are deep in the dermis, the mole has a bluish-black color and is called a "blue nevus."

The patient sheet deals with the benign melanocytic nevus. Our discussion will also be limited to a consideration of melanocytic nevi.

110

Diagnosis

The main problem is distinguishing a benign, growing nevus from a melanoma. It's common for worried patients to bring in their adolescent children because of rapid changes in their moles. Careful examination and explaining to the parents that moles normally grow and enlarge during this period usually suffice. One fact is invaluable: Malignant melanoma is practically unheard of before the age of 18 *except in congenital nevi*. With this in mind, it's almost always possible to reassure parents of a child or teen-ager regarding the usual melanocytic nevus.

In the adult, distinguishing between a benign melanocytic tumor—a nevus—and a malignant melanocytic tumor—a malignant melanoma—is a challenge. Survival of patients with melanoma depends on early diagnosis. If the criteria of a bleeding, nodular black mole are used to diagnose melanoma, it is usually too late. Melanomas can usually be diagnosed early by two findings that are rare in benign nevi:

1. Variegated coloration (Figure C-27). Be suspicious when you see red, white, or blue areas in a brown or black nevus.
2. An irregular border, often with angular induration or notches (Figures C-25 and C-26).

The clinical diagnosis of early melanoma, as well as its management, is the subject of an excellent recent review.[1]

Seborrheic keratoses (see Figure C-16), pigmented basal-cell carcinomas, skin tags, warts, and pyogenic granulomas are among the host of tumors that may resemble a melanocytic nevus. Don't be fooled by the small, deep hemangioma, which, because of its black color, can mimic a small melanoma. Firm thumb pressure on a hemangioma for one minute usually results in a significant color change resulting from expression of its blood content. If you're still worried, take a tiny punch biopsy. Often not recognized is the pigmented hairy *epidermal* nevus, or Becker's nevus, which is a pigmented patch that gradually enlarges and usually is first noticed in the late teens or early 20s. Microscopically the differentiation is obvious, since Becker's nevus does not contain nevus cells.

Treatment

The type of treatment depends on the reasons for having a mole removed. Is the mole unsightly? Is the patient concerned about malignancy? Does the physician suspect melanoma? Is the mole annoying because it protrudes?

Permanent eradication requires all the nevus cells to be destroyed or removed. This means full-thickness skin excision or destruction. Full-thickness skin excision provides an adequate sample for histology as well as ensuring removal of the mole. The resulting defect can be closed with sutures or, if small, may be allowed to heal by secondary intention using gelatin foam packing for hemostasis.

Partial, or shave, removal of a nevus is a useful technique for treating benign nevi that annoy because they protrude (Figures C-23 and C-24). Under local anesthesia, the protruding part of the nevus is removed with a blade or scissors, and a styptic applied to the wound. It's customary to submit the shaved-off portion for histology. This technique converts a protruding mole into a flat one. While there is almost always cosmetic improvement, it's rare that the mole becomes invisible. Tell this to your patients! Occasionally the mole becomes temporarily darker as a result of postsurgical inflammation.

Some physicians treat annoying nevi by shave removal—thus getting a sample for histology—followed by electrodesiccation of the wound base to destroy the remaining melanocytes. This occasionally gives magnificent results, but is unpredictable and, as with any electrodesiccation procedure, may leave a nasty scar. I don't use it. Of course, very *light* electrodesiccation for hemostasis following shave removal is a different matter, since it produces minimal scarring. Sole use of thermal destruction—by either cautery or electrodesiccation—is outmoded. It provides no specimen for histologic examination of suspicious lesions, and the resulting scarring is usually worse than that following cold steel surgery. Avoid cryotherapy, but for a different reason: It doesn't work. Nevi are amazingly resistant to liquid nitrogen freezing.

When to excise full thickness?

There is one clear-cut indication for full-thickness excision. If you strongly suspect malignancy, full-thickness excision should be performed as initial therapy and to provide the pathologist with an adequate specimen. The prognosis of melanoma—and consequently the type of therapy indicated—correlates closely with the depth of the lesion. The pathologist can only determine the prognosis from a full-thickness skin specimen. If your suspicion of melanoma is strong, infiltrate the anesthetic around the nevus and excise it with a small margin of normal tissue.

Although there are conflicting opinions about if and when to excise the common, ordinary-sized congenital nevus, full-thickness excision is the treatment of choice. If the patient is a child, wait until the early teens to ensure cooperation. Full-thickness excision is also a good approach when the patient is annoyed or concerned by one or two flat nevi and is not concerned about scarring.

When to shave-remove a nevus?

Shave or partial removal of a nevus is an efficient way of dealing with protuberant nevi that get nicked by razors or irritated by garments. Explain that you are simply removing the upper part of the mole and converting it to a flat mole. Nevi that are cosmetically annoying because they are protuberant can also be effectively dealt with by partial shave removal.

Shave surgery is a good way of dealing with a mole that concerns the patient but that you believe to be benign. This technique provides an adequate specimen for the pathologist to issue a reassuring report without the penalty of the significant scarring that usually results from full-thickness excision.

Shave removal is recommended only if you believe the lesion is benign; if you share your patient's concern about malignancy, do a full-thickness excision.

When to punch biopsy a nevus?

Rarely. The experienced clinician finds most nevi are best managed either by full-thickness excision or by shave surgery. When dealing with suspicious lesions in cosmetically sensitive areas, a preliminary punch biopsy may be wise. It's important to select the right portions of the nevus. Often it's best to take multiple small (1.5- to 2.0-mm) punches rather than one medium-sized punch. Punch biopsies have the advantage of providing the pathologist with a full-thickness skin specimen, but the drawback of sampling only a small portion of the nevus. Furthermore, surgical manipulation of a melanoma prior to complete excision is undesirable.

When to do nothing?

Often it's best to do nothing surgically. Parents read the cancer warning signs about a mole enlarging or changing color, become worried, and bring in their offspring for treatment. After careful examination, explain that we are continually growing new moles, and this normal process is especially rapid during adolescence. It saves time to have the parent read the patient instruction sheet on moles *after* you examine the child and pronounce the moles harmless, but *before* the question-and-answer period.

Sometimes it's prudent to modify the "don't treat" advice for nevi in children when the parents are very concerned. Snipping off a few nevi that worry the parents and submitting them for histologic examination may provide more reassurance than hours of explanation. Another challenge to the art of benign neglect is the child or young adult, frequently female, who wishes removal of all unsightly moles. Often descended from parents with many nevi, they wish to be spared a "moley" fate. Frequently they believe we possess some medical magic that will remove moles without a trace. "Don't treat" advice disappoints them and may raise doubts as to your ability. When careful explanation and the printed instruction sheet fail to convince, I refer patients to a conservative plastic surgeon for a second opinion.

Reference

1. Sober AJ, Fitzpatrick, TB, Mihm MC Jr: Primary melanoma of the skin: Recognition and management. *J Am Acad Dermatol* 2:179, 1980

25

Nickel allergy

Etiology

Allergy to nickel is common in women, occurring in about 10 per cent of Northern European and American women. Nickel contact dermatitis is usually caused by jewelry, but may also be produced by brassiere hooks, zippers, or the metal in eyeglass frames. In the pre-panty-hose days, thigh dermatitis from nickel-plated garter snaps was common. Persons allergic to nickel may get a rash wherever nickel-containing metal touches their skin. Curiously, nickel-containing coins infrequently cause dermatitis.

All jewelry contains nickel as a hardener, pure 24-karat gold being too soft for jewelry. There is less nickel in 14- or 18-karat gold jewelry than in inexpensive costume jewelry. Most women with weak nickel allergy who can't tolerate costume jewelry can wear jewelry made of 14- or 18-karat gold. Although stainless steel contains nickel, the nickel is tightly bound within the alloy and doesn't cause dermatitis. Therefore, patients with nickel allergy can handle stainless-steel articles provided they aren't nickel-plated.

Like other allergies, nickel allergy is acquired. Ear piercing sometimes initiates nickel allergy. Once nickel allergy appears, it persists for years.

Diagnosis

The history and distribution of the rash usually enable one to diagnose nickel contact dermatitis with confidence. When a woman tells you she breaks out from wearing costume jewelry, you can be certain she's allergic to nickel since nickel allergy is common in women. However, that doesn't necessarily mean that nickel caused the rash that's troubling her. It's the distribution of the rash—on the ear lobes, around the neck, on the back, under a ring—in a person with a history of nickel allergy that establishes the diagnosis of allergic contact dermatitis from nickel (Figures C-28 and C-29). Morphology isn't helpful, since nickel contact dermatitis resembles other processes such as atopic eczema, nummular eczema, and seborrheic dermatitis.

The presence of nickel allergy can be confirmed by patch testing.[1] Patch testing is superfluous in a patient with a typical history of breaking out from nickel-containing objects but may be of value in a patient with possible weak nickel allergy. Weak nickel allergy may cause an atypical dermatitis, such as recurrent crusting and oozing of the ear lobes, that's easy to misdiagnose as infection. Another diagnostic problem is recurring dermatitis underneath a ring without a history of dermatitis from other metal contact. Such ring dermatitis is usually not the result of nickel allergy, but represents the cumulative irritant effect of trapped detergents and moisture beneath the ring.

Treatment

When nickel allergy causes dermatitis, application of a topical corticosteroid and avoidance of further nickel contact usually clear up the rash. Patients with mild nickel allergy frequently tolerate 14- or 18-karat gold jewelry for limited periods of time. The prophylactic use of a topical corticosteroid when wearing jewelry is useful. For women whom nickel allergy prevents from wearing wedding rings, a compromise often works: They wear wedding rings only when away from home and apply a topical corticosteroid first.

Prevention

Preventing development of allergy to a widely used material is ordinarily impossible; however, nickel allergy presents one special situation—ear piercing. Tissue trauma facilitates sensitization. Nickel sensitization from ear piercing can be prevented by using hypoallergenic nickel-free earrings to maintain patency of the tracts until they heal. Special hypoallergenic stainless-steel ear-piercing kits and earrings are available from firms such as H&A Enterprises, Inc., 143-19 25th Avenue, Whitestone, N.Y. 11357.

Desensitization

At present there's no way to desensitize a person allergic to nickel. In some, the intensity of the allergy may spontaneously decrease over the years.

Managing the patient

Emphatically explain to your nickel-allergic patients that the only way to prevent dermatitis is to avoid skin contact with nickel-containing metals. Special stainless-steel hypoallergenic earrings are commercially available. Cloth padding can be inserted between nickel-plated zippers and brassiere hooks to prevent them from touching the skin. Plastic-covered rather than all-metal eyeglass frames should be worn. The fascinating subject of nickel allergy, as well as a useful "spot test" for determining which metal objects contain nickel, is covered superbly in Fisher's book.[1]

Reference

1. Fisher AA: *Contact Dermatitis,* 2nd edition. Philadelphia: Lea & Febiger, 1973

26

Pityriasis rosea

Etiology

Pityriasis rosea is a common, harmless disease of unknown cause. In its typical form a single scaly patch, the herald patch, precedes the generalized rash.

This generalized rash favors the trunk and spreads to the thighs, upper arms, and neck. Usually a few spots appear on the face, but they're rarely a cosmetic problem. The generalized eruption lasts for three to six weeks but occasionally disappears in a week or persists as long as three months. Mild malaise is common, significant systemic symptoms rare.

While most patients have few skin complaints, 10 to 20 per cent are uncomfortably itchy. Severe rashes resemble a florid drug eruption and are rare.

Diagnosis

Pityriasis rosea is commonly misdiagnosed by both patients and physicians as due to a fungus. When only the herald patch is present, microscopy of KOH-cleared skin scrapings may be necessary to exclude tinea corporis. The herald patch can also resemble eczema.

Once the typical generalized rash appears, it's clear that the condition is not tinea corporis, although it sometimes panics patients who believe their "fungus has spread." Secondary syphilis and a drug eruption are the main diagnostic problems. Check the mucous surfaces, palms, and soles, since they're favorite sites of secondary syphilis but are spared by pityriasis rosea. It's wise to order a serologic test for syphilis in adults. Pityriasis rosea may resemble any of the papulosquamous disorders—so add seborrheic dermatitis, tinea versicolor, and psoriasis to the bottom of your differential diagnostic list. Occasionally the rash "explodes" with myriads of macules that resemble measles or other viral exanthems.

Treatment

Most patients need only reassurance that their disease—although dramatic—is harmless and not contagious. Their mild skin irritability is minimized

116

by avoidance of soap and use of a lubricant. Skin lubrication is readily accomplished with bath oils.

When itching makes the patient uncomfortable, corticosteroids should be used. While most textbooks recommend topical corticosteroids, they're relatively ineffective. A 10- to 14-day tapering course of systemic corticosteroids usually produces a dramatic improvement in symptoms. Prednisone is the preferred steroid and should be given as a single morning dose. I use a regimen similar to the one for poison oak/poison ivy and start with 40 to 60 mg the first day, decreasing the dosage by 5 mg per day. Sometimes a second course is necessary.

Tell the patient the prednisone is for comfort and is not a cure. Before starting prednisone inquire about peptic ulcers, diabetes, hypertension, and asthma—although these are only relative contraindications. Since concern about side effects of corticosteroids is common (and well-founded), explain that this applies generally to long-term therapy, not to the two-week course you are prescribing.

Ultraviolet light therapy shortens the course of pityriasis rosea. However, the cost and nuisance of multiple ultraviolet light treatments are seldom justified in this disease. During warm weather you may wish to tell patients that moderate sun exposure several times a week will speed healing.

The main treatment is reassurance. Fear of contagion, concern about scarring, and worry about diet are anxieties that a few words—and the patient information sheet—should put to rest.

Poison ivy/poison oak (*Rhus* allergy)

27

Etiology

Acute contact dermatitis in North America from poison ivy (East and Midwest) or poison oak (West) is exceedingly common. Poison ivy/oak dermatitis is an example of allergic contact dermatitis. Its common occurrence and frequent severity merit a separate patient instruction sheet. The allergens in poison ivy, poison oak, and poison sumac are similar, and the clinical manifestations and treatment are essentially identical. These plants all belong to the genus *Rhus*.

Rhus dermatitis results from skin contact with the plants' oleoresins. The patient may have come into either direct contact with the plant or indirect contact with the oleoresin, which can be carried on the fur of a pet, on clothing or hands, or via smoke. The allergen is not spread by wind or air.

Diagnosis

The diagnosis in most cases is easy; usually patients have correctly made their own diagnosis and desire treatment. Irregular patches and streaks of acute contact dermatitis (Figure C-30) point to a plant, and in North America that plant is almost always *Rhus*. A history of a recent outing in areas known to be infested with *Rhus* increases the likelihood that the diagnosis is correct. Other plants, such as *Primula obconica* and Algerian ivy, can cause plant contact dermatitis morphologically indistinguishable from *Rhus* dermatitis. Usually one diagnoses *Rhus* dermatitis when confronted with a plant contact dermatitis and a history of probable exposure. It helps when the patient knows he's allergic to *Rhus* plants. Patch testing with *Rhus* allergen is not helpful.

Diagnosing *Rhus* dermatitis can be difficult when the contact was indirect—through a pet, clothing, or some other object—even the patient's own skin. Such skin-to-skin transfer is not uncommon in male patients who develop genital dermatitis from transfer of oleoresin from hands to penis while urinating. Indirect plant contact dermatitis doesn't have the streaky, sharp-

118

ly demarcated patches that suggest plant contact, but consists of diffuse areas of dermatitis. Diagnosing *Rhus* dermatitis caused by indirect contact may require considerable questioning and detective work; sometimes a correct diagnosis can be made only after repeated bouts of dermatitis.

Treatment

Treatment of *Rhus* dermatitis consists of suppression with corticosteroids. Corticosteroids provide dramatic relief. Unfortunately, preventing future episodes of contact dermatitis is difficult. Be sure the patient knows the plants' appearance; pictures help, but the best approach is to have a friend or neighbor point out the troublemaker. Poison ivy can be a low, creeping plant or a climbing vine; poison oak is a bush that can grow over six feet high.

Washing after *Rhus* exposure is a time-honored preventive measure. Unfortunately, it's seldom effective. The allergen is rapidly bound to the skin; in order to prevent dermatitis, it's necessary to wash within 15 minutes of contact. Washing does rapidly destroy the oleoresin, and washing garments or an exposed pet will prevent the indirect spread of oleoresin. Strong soaps and detergents are unnecessary, since the *Rhus* allergen is unstable in the presence of moisture.

Desensitization as a method of preventing *Rhus* dermatitis remains an unrealized dream. Most preparations designed to "desensitize" are inactive and without value. Potent *Rhus* extract, available from Hollister-Stier Laboratories, temporarily decreases sensitivity to *Rhus* plants. When the "desensitization" treatments are stopped, the sensitivity usually returns to its previous level. Furthermore, such treatment may cause side effects. I haven't attempted to "desensitize" patients to *Rhus* for 15 years; it's simpler to treat acute episodes with a short course of systemic corticosteroids.

Specific therapy of acute *Rhus* dermatitis

Systemic corticosteroids work quickly and can prevent the weeks of blistering and misery that severe *Rhus* dermatitis causes. Systemic corticosteroids are essential in the acute phase, since topical corticosteroids can't penetrate the swollen, blistered skin. Use enough corticosteroid to suppress the eruption. Usually 60 to 100 mg of prednisone a day are adequate; severe cases may initially require daily doses of 200 mg. As the dermatitis improves, the daily amount of corticosteroid is reduced. A 10- to 14-day course of oral steroids usually suffices.

Prednisone is the preferred corticosteroid. In mild to moderate *Rhus* dermatitis it's best taken as a single morning dose. In severe contact dermatitis, when doses of more than 100 mg are required, have the patient divide his daily dose and take half in the morning and half in the evening. The prednisone schedule I use for treating moderately severe *Rhus* contact dermatitis is given in Table 27-1. Prescribing 20-mg prednisone tablets, rather than the usual 5-mg tablets, may lessen patients' concerns about taking high doses.

What's "enough" corticosteroid? Treatment must be individualized, especially for severe cases. When enough is prescribed, the patient should im-

TABLE 27-1

Schedule for treating moderately severe *Rhus* dermatitis with prednisone tablets as a single morning dose

DAY	PREDNISONE MG	DOSE NO. OF 20-MG TABLETS
1	80	4
2	70	3½
3	60	3
4	50	2½
5	40	2
6	40	2
7	30	1½
8	30	1¹/₂
9	20	1
10	20	1
11	10	½
12	10	½
13	0	0

prove daily. Tell the patient to call you if he fails to improve each day. The occasional patient who fails to improve day by day is instructed to take extra prednisone for a few days. In the early stages of *Rhus* contact dermatitis it's impossible to determine whether the attack is going to be relatively mild or severe. When treating patients whose history of repeated severe attacks of *Rhus* contact dermatitis suggests a high degree of allergy, it's wise to initiate treatment with more than the usual amount of corticosteroid.

Systemic corticosteroid therapy can be provided in other ways than oral prednisone. Some physicians use injections of ACTH; others inject repository corticosteroids. Injection of long-acting repository steroids such as triamcinolone acetonide should be avoided, since they remain in the patient's body much longer than necessary. In addition to oral prednisone, I frequently inject 4 mg of dexamethasone phosphate intramuscularly at the initial visit. This rapidly acting, soluble corticosteroid provides the patient an immediate systemic effect and the psychological boost of having something done for him at once.

The safety of such short courses of systemic corticosteroids has been documented and is attested to by their almost universal use in treating *Rhus* dermatitis in North America. Active peptic ulcers, while not an absolute contraindication, suggest caution and the briefest possible course of corticosteroids. Mood-altering effects occur occasionally, but are rarely severe. Diabetics should be warned that corticosteroids may worsen their disease.

The major problem with short courses of systemic corticosteroids is patient concern. Most patients have heard horror stories of persons whose "health

Poison ivy/poison oak

was ruined by cortisone." Head this off by emphasizing that short courses of corticosteroids are safe (after all, the body makes cortisone); it's prolonged steroid intake over months or years that produces dangerous side effects. For persons who suffer frequent bouts of *Rhus* dermatitis, as many as four courses annually can safely be prescribed. Each time I warn the patient to take all precautions to avoid future episodes of *Rhus* dermatitis.

Should one prescribe a supply of prednisone for patients who unavoidably now and then get severe *Rhus* dermatitis? I do this only for a few reliable patients whose occupations or avocations make it unavoidable.

Other systemic drugs such as antihistamines, sedatives, or tranquilizers are unnecessary in treating *Rhus* contact dermatitis. Antihistamines don't suppress contact dermatitis, nor are they antipruritic except for their sedative side effects. When *Rhus* contact dermatitis is adequately controlled by systemic corticosteroids, sedation is unnecessary. There are always exceptions. Occasionally, when there's severe itching and distress, patients are grateful for two or three days of bedtime hydroxyzine or a similar nonbarbiturate sedative.

Topical therapy

During the acute, swollen, vesicular stage, what the patient doesn't apply to his skin is more important than what he does. Topical therapy doesn't help at this stage. The wrong topical may even aggravate the dermatitis, since anesthetic ointments can sensitize, alcohol and astringents may irritate, and calamine and other lotions make a mess without doing much good. Cool compresses are soothing and help remove debris and crusts. While water is as good as anything, patients will be more impressed if one or two tablespoons of ordinary white vinegar are added to each quart of cool water. Burow's solution, saline, or similar bland liquids will do as well. Once the blisters and crusts have cleared up, the compresses should be stopped and topical corticosteroids begun.

Subacute poison-oak contact dermatitis is helped by topical corticosteroids. Any one of the medium-potency corticosteroids (Chapter 1) will do nicely. Most patients prefer a cream formulation. CAUTION: **Corticosteroid creams containing a high percentage of propylene glycol may irritate and should be avoided.**

Patients may bathe as desired but are told not to apply soap to the rash, since soap is an irritant. Dry skin may be annoying in the later stages; if this occurs, have the patient lubricate it as suggested in the dry-skin dermatitis patient instructions.

Complications

Practically none. Mild corticosteroid side effects occur occasionally—stomach and abdominal pain and slight mood changes, especially insomnia and jitteriness. If gastrointestinal problems arise, add antacids and taper off the prednisone quickly. Reassurance is all that's needed for mild mood alterations; in the rare patient with drastic psychic changes, stop the corticosteroids at once.

Remember that corticosteroid side effects bear more relation to the length of treatment than to the amount of drug: It's safer to take 200 mg of prednisone in one day than 10 mg daily for 20 days. Too often one encounters patients who have been itching, blistering, and unable to go to work or school for weeks because of inadequate doses of systemic corticosteroids.

Pyoderma is an unusual complication of *Rhus* contact dermatitis. Secondary infection is an indication for treatment with systemic antibiotics; erythromycin or a semisynthetic penicillin is a good choice.

Poison ivy/poison oak

28

Postoperative care

Postoperative care instruction sheets save you time; you'll receive fewer telephone calls from anxious patients and be spared answering the same questions umpteen times. The methods described here are effective and can be modified for special cases. For example, you may want to keep a sutured wound dry longer than the two days advised in the patient sheet.

Skin surgery leaves a wound that either is closed with sutures or remains as an open defect that gradually epithelializes. Postoperative care following open surgery differs from care after closed surgery; they're discussed separately. A third section covers care after liquid nitrogen destruction.

Do wounds heal better dry than wet? Tradition holds that a dry crust is desirable, as it protects the wound and discourages infection. Recent studies, however, have shown that wounds epithelialize faster if occluded to prevent loss of moisture and drying of the surface. Crusts retard healing by acting as a mechanical barrier to the regenerating epidermis. "Moist" postoperative care aims to prevent crust formation by using ointments and/or occlusive dressings to keep the wound from drying out.

The moist technique is also useful for sutured wounds. Epithelium needs to fill the gap between the sutured wound edges—and it does so more rapidly if the wound is occluded to prevent desiccation.

Open wounds

Should your patients use the dry or the wet approach for caring for open wounds? I use both. The dry technique is simple and usually works as well as the moist technique, with its more cumbersome bandage and ointment. Most open wounds following superficial dermatologic surgery are covered with a crust that results from the use of a styptic such as Monsel's solution. Styptics should be used only on superficial wounds. If deep wounds are left open, use gelatin foam and/or pressure to control bleeding.

The moist postoperative technique should be employed when optimal cosmetic results are important. Superficial wounds without crusts and any deep open wounds are better managed by the moist postoperative technique.

123

Dry technique

Use the instruction sheet titled "Care After Superficial Skin Surgery." The patient is asked to ignore the wound except for painting the crust twice daily with ordinary rubbing alcohol. Alcohol applications decrease bacterial colonization and are something innocuous that patients can put on their wounds—otherwise they're tempted to apply their own "healing" potions.

Moist technique

Use the instruction sheet titled "Wound Care." Occlusion is achieved with an ointment and a bandage. It isn't as perfect as occlusion achieved by covering the wound with plastic film, but represents a practical compromise. Some physicians prefer an antibiotic ointment to discourage bacterial growth; there's no proof that this is superior to petrolatum (Vaseline). Ideally the moist technique should be used until the wound has epithelialized. The wound care directions are a compromise between moist and dry healing and allow the patient to leave the wound open after a firm crust has formed, reducing the time a bandage is needed. You may wish to modify the wound care sheet to continue occlusion until healing is complete.

The wound care sheet is used when wounds have been *partially* closed with sutures. Partial wound closure should be explained to patients so they understand that you left the wound partially open on purpose and not by mistake.

Closed surgery

A separate instruction sheet details care of the sutured wound. Initially an ointment and bandage are used to prevent desiccation and crust formation, which interfere with epithelialization.

To avoid "railroad-track" scarring, I remove sutures early and then apply a tape wound support to prevent dehiscence and minimize scar spreading. I currently use flesh-colored "paper" tape (Micropore) applied over spirit gum adhesive. Hollister medical adhesive is an alternative to spirit gum.

This tape support system sticks tenaciously for over a week in most locations. It won't loosen with water, and patients are glad to be able to bathe as usual. The system isn't sterile, but sterility isn't necessary at this point. Tape wound supports are not practical in hairy areas. Even on a closely shaved beard, a few days' growth loosens tape. On hairy skin I apply flexible collodion directly to the wound as a support. The collodion is shed in a few days. Although not as good as tape support, it's better than nothing.

When gut is used for wound closure (Chapter 3), use the "Care of Wounds Closed With Dissolving Stitches" instruction sheet. This sheet explains that the sutures will be shed spontaneously and need not be removed.

Liquid nitrogen instructions

The liquid nitrogen instruction sheet differs from the other postoperative instructions in that it discusses liquid nitrogen treatment and follow-up care. Patients may be unfamiliar with liquid nitrogen treatment. I explain that (1) the mild pain lasts only a few minutes and (2) the growth is intact after freezing and will be shed later on.

When freezing lesions deeply, stress that marked blistering can occur and is part of the treatment, *not* a complication. Patients are sometimes frightened by pronounced eyelid swelling following liquid nitrogen treatment about the eyelids. Alert patients to the possibility of marked swelling when lesions about the eyelids are treated. Reassure them that this will disappear by itself over a few days.

Liquid nitrogen treatment frees the patient from worry about follow-up care. The wound almost invariably heals nicely irrespective of what the patient does. The liquid nitrogen instruction sheet doesn't mention infection as a possible complication, as infection is rare following the superficial liquid nitrogen freezing used in treating benign lesions.

The last paragraph asks the patient to return if liquid nitrogen treatment doesn't eradicate his lesion. I reinforce this instruction when talking with the patient. Why? Liquid nitrogen is used on lesions clinically diagnosed as benign, but sometimes we err. Diagnostic error is a particular problem in freezing actinic keratoses, since a skin cancer may mimic a benign keratosis. Biopsy any keratosis that fails to respond to liquid nitrogen. These concerns about recurring lesions don't apply to recurrence of typical warts—unhappily a frequent event.

Pruritus ani (rectal itch)

29

Etiology

Pruritus ani is common in North America; because of their embarrassment, its victims often admit they have it only after direct questioning. As a result of popular advertising for hemorrhoid preparations, patients frequently attribute their anal itching to hemorrhoids although they may not have these nuisances. Hemorrhoids themselves don't itch; sometimes, when numerous, hemorrhoids cause retention of fecal material, and this causes anal itching.

Diagnosis

In most patients pruritus ani has no obvious cause. Although some texts state that diseases of the anal canal cause pruritus ani, cases that result from anal disease are distinctly unusual. Of the specific causes of pruritus ani, psoriasis is the most common. Dermatitis of the perianal skin occurs frequently in psoriasis, characteristically with extension into the gluteal cleft. All patients complaining of pruritus ani should be thoroughly examined for psoriasis. Psoriatic involvement of other skin areas may be minimal, and only some pitting of the fingernails or a scaly plaque on the scalp, elbows, or knees will lead to the correct diagnosis. Not infrequently pruritus ani appears to be a forme fruste of psoriasis.

Fungal infection is a less frequent cause of pruritus ani. It's more common in males and frequently is associated with tinea cruris with sharply demarcated scaly patches of the inner thighs. Fungal infections usually extend well onto the skin of the buttocks, whereas idiopathic pruritus ani is limited to the immediate perianal skin. Candidiasis, with its macerated skin, superficial erosions, and satellite lesions, may sometimes be superimposed on idiopathic pruritus ani.

In the majority of patients with "idiopathic" pruritus ani two factors play an etiologic role: (1) the irritant effects of the stool and (2) the relative irritability of the perianal skin. Stools are irritating to skin; witness the inflammation produced in babies or incontinent adults when fecal matter isn't

126

promptly cleaned from perianal skin. Most persons, however, while having experienced transient irritation from stools, do not complain of pruritus ani. Patients with pruritus ani have unusually sensitive, easily irritated perianal skin. Many patients with pruritus ani show additional signs of skin dysfunction—for example, hand dermatitis, otitis externa, or seborrheic dermatitis of the scalp.

Treatment

Specific

In the relatively few cases when a specific cause can be found, treatment is directed at the cause. Dermatophyte infestations respond well to one of the newer, less irritating antifungal creams such as haloprogin (Halotex), miconazole (Monistat), or clotrimazole (Lotrimin, Mycelex). Psoriasis of the anal area and gluteal cleft responds to 1 to 2 per cent hydrocortisone applied sparingly two or three times daily. In most patients with pruritus ani, therapy must be aimed at soothing the perianal skin and reducing irritation.

Minimizing irritation

Reducing the irritant effects of stools with careful anal hygiene is the most important step in treating idiopathic pruritus ani. Cleansing after bowel movements must be meticulous and gentle and is best accomplished with water. European authors often advise using a bidet—a measure hardly practical in North America. Some patients—especially those with much perianal hair—find it necessary to shower for adequate post-bowel-movement cleansing. Dry toilet paper *must* be avoided. A reasonable compromise is to use moist toilet paper gently until all traces of stool are gone, then blot the area gently with dry toilet paper. Moistened, foil-wrapped tissues designed for anal cleansing are commercially available. While useful for the traveler, they're more expensive than water-moistened toilet paper and occasionally their alcohol content irritates. A spray of water from a rubber-bulb syringe may prove useful for patients in whom hemorrhoids, excessive hair, or tender skin renders moist toilet paper ineffective for proper anal cleansing.

Diarrhea, fecal leakage, and mucoid discharge all aggravate pruritus ani by exposing the perianal skin to irritant bowel contents. Sometimes the diarrhea is caused by an antibiotic. Chronic diarrhea is an indication for help from a consultant. Fecal leakage is occasionally the result of anal-canal disease such as fissures or cryptitis. Pruritus ani is rarely relieved by elimination of anal-canal disease or other proctologic procedures.

In some persons certain foods, especially coffee and spicy dishes, induce gastrointestinal hyperactivity with increased bowel movements and mucoid anal discharge. Eliminating the foods responsible for the bowel irritability may be dramatically effective. Not much can be done to relieve pruritus ani in patients with slight sphincter incontinence and frequent flatus. One approach is to keep a pledget of cotton outside the anus, held in place by the buttocks, to absorb anything expelled per anum. Commercial nonwoven fabric patches cut especially for this purpose (Tucks) are available.

The patient instruction sheet stresses the role of gentle, careful anal hygiene. Scrubbing with soap and water is an almost universal response to itching. Soap is irritating; it should never be used on the perianal skin, since plain water does an adequate job. The instructions prohibit self-treatment with proprietary anti-itch remedies, which can irritate the skin.

Topicals

Topical corticosteroids, when properly used, are effective. Only hydrocortisone-containing topicals should be employed; the fluorinated corticosteroids interfere with cell replication and may cause skin thinning with disastrous consequences. If possible, try to control the pruritus with 1 per cent hydrocortisone cream. Higher hydrocortisone concentrations such as 2 or 3 per cent, while more effective, carry the risk of skin thinning (see Chapter 1). Patients should apply the hydrocortisone topical sparingly with a fingertip after bowel movements, at bedtime, and possibly once or twice more every day. As the dermatitis improves, the topical corticosteroid can be used less and less. The relapse rate after successful treatment of pruritus ani is high; recurrences usually yield to a repetition of the original regimen.

WARNING: **Topical medicaments frequently irritate perianal skin.** Even topical corticosteroids may irritate and aggravate pruritus ani. Be wary of irritation and avoid potential sensitizers such as topical anesthetics.

Systemic therapy

When there is severe perianal dermatitis, especially with a superimposed allergic contact dermatitis from a topical medicament, a brief course of systemic corticosteroids is indicated. Usually prednisone taken for 7 to 14 days as a gradually decreasing daily morning dose suffices. Sometimes pruritus ani requires longer periods of a systemic corticosteroid for control. This is a problem mainly when previous therapy with fluorinated corticosteroids has resulted in a thin, extremely irritable perianal skin not responsive to topical hydrocortisone. When confronted with this dilemma, I usually initiate a three- to six-week course of alternate-day prednisone. Some of my colleagues prefer periodic ACTH injections. Tell your patient that the systemic corticosteroid therapy is a temporary measure to provide some relief while his skin recovers sufficiently for control by topical medication.

Some physicians view pruritus ani as a psychosomatic illness and are fond of prescribing sedatives for it. The pruritus ani is allegedly part of a compulsive, perfectionistic personality. Although some pruritus ani patients are preoccupied with anal hygiene, the majority have objective evidence of other skin abnormalities, and a psychosomatic explanation does them injustice. At any rate, from the standpoint of therapy the question of psychosomatic causation of pruritus ani is moot. A patient's personality won't change with counseling and sedatives. With proper dermatologic care, most patients get relief.

30

Psoriasis

Etiology

Psoriasis is a curse to patient and physician. Textbooks invariably—and appropriately—describe it as a chronic dermatitis. In spite of intensive research, we know little more than that psoriasis involves excessively rapid turnover of epidermal cells. Psoriasis is an inherited disorder; the genetic mechanism is complex.

Diagnosis

Diagnosis of the classical presentation—sharply demarcated, scaling plaques of the scalp, elbows, and knees—is easy, but psoriasis can appear in ways that baffle even the most experienced clinician. Psoriasis may present difficulties when it affects only the palms (Figure C-31), soles, or fingernails (Figure C-34). Psoriasis may begin insidiously and initially resemble such disorders as seborrheic dermatitis, nummular eczema, dry-skin dermatitis, atopic eczema, or hand dermatitis (Figures C-31, C-32, and C-33). Most dermatologists have learned to view with suspicion stubborn seborrheic dermatitis of the scalp; years later, it often develops into classical psoriasis.

Treatment

Psoriasis affects between 1.5 and 3 per cent of the Caucasian population and thus represents an important therapeutic challenge. Patients with newly developed psoriasis often become disenchanted with their treatment and switch physicians in the hope of finding a cure. While we still lack a cure, treatment usually offers significant temporary relief and sometimes clears up the rash.

Since psoriasis is a disorder requiring long-term treatment, therapy should be simple and inexpensive.

The effective, currently available treatment modalities for psoriasis are listed in Table 30-1. More than 90 per cent of psoriatics require only topical

TABLE 30-1

Treatment modalities for psoriasis

Topical therapy
    Corticosteroids
    Tar
    Anthralin
Intralesional injections of corticosteroids
Sunlight
Ultraviolet light
    Alone
    With topical potentiation
    With systemic potentiation (PUVA therapy)
Systemic
X-ray

---

therapy. Systemic therapy is the therapy of desperation and should be reserved for patients whose severe psoriasis fails to respond to topicals.

The patient information sheet on psoriasis contains mainly background information and hammers home the theme that the aim of treatment is control rather than cure. Since the treatment of psoriasis varies with severity and location of disease, routine printed treatment instructions are not feasible. Since treatment is often complicated, it's wise to write out specific treatment instructions for each patient.

Topical therapy

The topicals used for psoriasis are corticosteroids, tars, and anthralin, in addition to a few miscellaneous agents of limited usefulness such as salicylic acid and phenol. Topical mercurials, while once popular, have fallen into disfavor, as occasional toxicity has resulted. Avoid them.

Corticosteroids are the most popular topicals; they neither stain nor stink. Major disadvantage? The control they achieve is usually transient, and daily applications are generally needed. In certain areas atrophy from the more potent fluorinated corticosteroids becomes a limiting factor. They are expensive. There is a considerable difference in the efficacy of fluorinated corticosteroids in psoriasis.

Tars are some of the better agents for treating psoriasis. In the United States, chiefly coal tars are used in treating psoriasis; wood tars are preferred by some. All tars stain and have a characteristic odor. Coal tar is a potent photosensitizer. Both coal and wood tars occasionally produce allergic sensitization and a resulting contact dermatitis. Traditionally coal tar was used compounded in petrolatum—an effective but messy preparation.

There are numerous proprietary coal-tar preparations in the forms of lotions, creams, gels, or tar-oil bath additives. Proprietary tar preparations are less messy and less expensive than tar ointments compounded to order. Ev-

Psoriasis

ery dermatologist has his favorites.* Coal-tar solution is a solubilized fraction of coal tar that can be used diluted to 25 per cent in alcohol as a scalp tincture or added at 5 to 10 per cent to a corticosteroid cream.

Anthralin is an effective but hard-to-use topical because it's irritating and, if not used cautiously, may worsen psoriasis. It can stain clothing permanently. Fluorinated corticosteroids increase the irritating effect of anthralin and should not be used with it. Patients should have stopped fluorinated corticosteroid topicals for a month before starting anthralin.

In spite of these drawbacks, anthralin is a valuable preparation. When used judiciously, it can work wonders on extensive body psoriasis. My preference is for anthralin in ointment form, marketed in the United States as Anthra-Derm in 0.1, 0.25, 0.5, and 1.0 per cent concentrations. Start with the 0.1 per cent concentration and have the patient apply it precisely and sparingly at bedtime to a test area. If tolerated in the test area, it can be applied to the remaining areas. Demonstrate how to apply a microscopically thin film of the ointment and then massage it in well. After applying the ointment, the patient must wash his hands, as anthralin is irritating to the eyes. If the 0.1 per cent concentration is tolerated, this strength is used nightly until no further benefit is obtained; then the concentration is increased to 0.25 per cent. Later on, depending on the response, the concentration may be increased further. If you use anthralin: (1) be cautious, as it's irritating, (2) don't use fluorinated corticosteroids at the same time, and (3) warn the patient that it can stain clothing permanently. The last problem can be minimized by applying the ointment at bedtime and bathing in the morning.

In psoriasis, the response to topical medications shows striking regional variations. Medications useful in the groin and armpits will have no effect on scalp psoriasis, while topicals designed for scalp psoriasis are usually too irritating to be used in skin-fold areas. This variation in response accounts for the complexity of topical therapy.

Scalp
1. The patient should shampoo daily, if possible. This is to remove the continuous accumulation of scale. The type of shampoo the patient uses makes little difference. Medicated shampoos are not effective against psoriasis.
2. A coal-tar preparation should be applied sparingly to the psoriatic areas three to 12 hours before each shampoo. By applying it sparingly and precisely, the patient can minimize the smell and staining. Tar-oil bath additives, or coal-tar solution 10 to 20 per cent in alcohol, can be painted sparingly with a cotton-tipped applicator on psoriatic patches (preferably by someone other than the patient). Tar gels are good alternatives that patients can easily apply themselves.
3. Topical corticosteroids—solutions, lotions, or gels—work well on scalp margins but are of less benefit on the hairy scalp. (Creams and ointments are

---

*Some over-the-counter preparations are Alphosyl and Tar-Doak (lotions and creams), Psorigel and Estar Gel (gels), and Balnetar and Doak Oil (tar-oil combinations). The tar-oil combinations, while marketed as bath additives, are useful when painted directly on the skin.

hard to apply to the scalp and should be avoided.) Hydrocortisone has little impact on psoriasis of the scalp; a fluorinated corticosteroid should be used. Unfortunately, the fluorinated corticosteroid lotions and gels are expensive. Less expensive lotions can be made by mixing many of the fluorinated corticosteroid creams with three or four times their volume of water.

4. Anthralin hair pomades and liquids are effective but are tricky to use, as anthralin may irritate. Anthralin stains hair, clothing, and skin.

Ears and scalp edges

Fluorinated corticosteroid creams, gels, and ointments usually nicely suppress psoriasis of the ears and scalp edges. Surprisingly often, patients prefer ointments. If used sparingly at bedtime, ointments are cosmetically acceptable. Psoriasis of the ear canals can be very stubborn; a concentrated corticosteroid ointment applied thinly once or twice daily with fingertip or cotton-tipped applicator usually suppresses it. In some persons, ear psoriasis is prone to repeated infections, which are often treated as "chronically infected otitis externa" by nondermatologists (Figure C-36). Vigorous treatment of the ear-canal psoriasis with topical corticosteroids generally prevents such episodes. Sometimes a tetracycline-corticosteroid (Terra-Cortril) or erythromycin-corticosteroid topical combination is useful when steroids alone are inadequate.

Face

When psoriasis involves the face, it's generally mild. A cream containing 2 to 3 per cent hydrocortisone applied sparingly twice daily usually controls it. If this doesn't suffice, add 2 per cent sulfur and 2 per cent salicylic acid to the hydrocortisone topical. Avoid fluorinated corticosteroids on the face; they may cause rosaceaform eruptions as well as atrophy with telangiectasia.

Skin folds

Psoriasis of the armpits, groin (Figure C-37), and perianal skin must be treated differently from lesions elsewhere. These skin folds are sensitive to traditional remedies such as anthralin and tars, which often irritate, and to the fluorinated corticosteroids, which may cause skin thinning and atrophy. Perianal involvement in psoriasis is common. The most frequent cause of pruritus ani is mild, often unrecognized psoriasis (Figure C-35). Gentle skin care is essential in perianal psoriasis. Hand the patient the pruritus ani patient instructions. Start the patient on 1 per cent hydrocortisone cream applied very thinly two or three times a day and instruct him to use it less often when there is improvement.

Psoriasis of the inguinal folds and armpits should be treated similarly to psoriasis of the gluteal cleft, by avoiding irritants and using hydrocortisone topically. Patients should be instructed to avoid soap in these areas—something they don't like. Deodorants are irritating to many patients with armpit psoriasis. Suggest either a drying powder as a deodorant, or a neomycin-containing cream. If the latter is used, warn the patient that it might cause a sensitivity reaction.

What if 1 per cent hydrocortisone doesn't work? Increase the concentration of hydrocortisone to 2 to 3 per cent. This will control the majority of rashes. Patients using 2 to 3 per cent hydrocortisone topicals should taper them off as soon as they're better.

Do not use fluorinated corticosteroids in the armpits, groin, or perianal area. While often dramatically effective over the short term, they tend to cause thinning and atrophy, with resulting irritable, hypersensitive skin. The patient uses the fluorinated steroid more and more, the skin gets thinner and thinner, and the rash gets steadily worse. It often takes months to reverse the atrophy produced by just a few weeks of fluorinated corticosteroids. Even 2 to 3 per cent hydrocortisone occasionally causes skin thinning in skin-fold areas.

Body, arms, and legs
1. Fluorinated corticosteroids are the simplest therapy for psoriasis of these areas and suffice in many patients. However, when there is extensive psoriasis, one must consider both the cost of these preparations and the degree of systemic absorption. Corticosteroids used in psoriasis tend to produce a temporary effect; relapse usually occurs within days of stopping them. The effect of corticosteroids can be greatly accentuated by occluding them with plastic film for three to eight hours each day as described in Chapter 1.
2. Coal tar is a traditional remedy for body psoriasis. Although it stains and has an odor, it's often effective. For mild to moderate body psoriasis, try combining coal tar applied at bedtime with a fluorinated corticosteroid applied sparingly in the morning. The patient may wish to use old pajamas and sheets and remove any remaining tar with a morning shower.
3. The use of anthralin ointment is described above.

Hands
Psoriasis of the hands (Figures C-31, C-32, and C-33) is best treated with topical corticosteroids according to the location and severity of the dermatitis. Details are given in the unit on hand dermatitis. Most often treatment with potent fluorinated corticosteroids and plastic occlusion will be necessary. Remember that this can cause skin thinning, so use it carefully. Psoriasis of the hands may be a difficult therapeutic challenge.

Feet
Psoriasis of the feet tends to involve the soles, often with formation of deep-set vesicles and pustules. Potent fluorinated corticosteroids applied at bedtime and covered overnight with plastic are the most effective therapy of psoriasis of the soles. Plastic occlusion of the feet is best accomplished by using a small plastic bag (the type available in grocery stores for food storage) cut down and held in place with a sock overnight. As an alternative, use Saran Wrap or similar plastic food wrap held in place with a sock. Cautions regarding skin thinning with this treatment apply to the soles as well as the

hands. As the patient improves, he should use the treatment less often. Friction markedly aggravates psoriasis; patients with psoriasis of the feet should be encouraged to wear shoes and socks and avoid going barefoot, especially on rough surfaces.

Intralesional therapy

Intralesional injection of repository corticosteroids is a practical approach to limited areas of psoriasis—especially for the patient who has cosmetically annoying psoriasis of the elbows and knees. For psoriasis, use triamcinolone acetonide suspension 10 mg/ml (Kenalog-10) injected at a depth of 3 to 7 mm as described in Chapter 1.

Sunlight

Most psoriatics are improved by sunlight. Sunburn should be avoided as it—like any other skin injury—may aggravate psoriasis. If coal tar is used, caution patients that tar is a potent photosensitizer. I encourage those patients who benefit from sunlight to take sunbaths two or three times a week when possible. The face should be protected with a sunscreen; the benefits of sun must be weighed against its skin-damaging effects.

Ultraviolet light

Short-wave "sunburn" ultraviolet light, termed ultraviolet B (UV-B), is of modest benefit in psoriasis. The traditional hot quartz mercury lamps, as well as the fluorescent sun bulbs, emit UV-B. The effectiveness of UV-B is potentiated by coal tar. Systematic use of coal tar and ultraviolet light, termed the Goeckerman treatment, is an effective although rather involved way of treating extensive psoriasis.

Long-wave ultraviolet light, ultraviolet A (UV-A), is of little value by itself. However, when psoralens are used as photoactivators with UV-A, it's a powerful new tool in the treatment of psoriasis. Treatment with oral psoralens and UV-A light (named PUVA = Psoralen + UV-A) is a very effective treatment for severe, extensive psoriasis. Both special light sources and special expertise are required.

Stable versus unstable psoriasis

The traditional therapy of psoriasis applies to stable psoriasis—scaly, hyperkeratotic patches present for months or years. At times psoriasis becomes unstable and spreads rapidly. When this happens, traditional treatments must be stopped. Unstable, spreading, irritable psoriasis is made worse by the strong tar or anthralin remedies often necessary to subdue chronic psoriasis.

Treat unstable psoriasis with utmost caution and gentleness. Lubrication and topical corticosteroids in nonirritating vehicles are your best bet, possibly augmented by mild tars or low-dose ultraviolet light. With time, unstable psoriasis usually becomes stable and then responds to traditional antipsoriatic remedies.

Why this caution? Unstable psoriasis is markedly irritable and prone to aggravation by inappropriate therapy. Strong remedies not only worsen unstable psoriasis and cause additional lesions, but may lead to exfoliative dermatitis. Warn the patient that his skin is sensitive; he must avoid anything that irritates, and he is likely to get worse before getting better. Resist the temptation to use potent antipsoriatic remedies in the face of rapidly spreading psoriasis.

What causes psoriasis to become unstable and spread? Streptococcal pharyngitis is a well-documented triggering factor, especially in the young. The resulting droplike showers of new psoriatic lesions (guttate psoriasis) usually respond nicely to mild treatment over a period of months. Other types of physical stress—infections, injuries, or surgery—may cause psoriasis to become destabilized. A severe sunburn, irritating topical therapy, unrelated contact dermatitis (poison ivy, poison oak), or similar skin insult may activate psoriasis. Often the cause of psoriatic instability is unknown. Whatever the cause, it's important to recognize psoriatic instability and suitably modify treatment.

Systemic treatment

Antimetabolites

Antimetabolites have been used with success in psoriasis. These cellular poisons reduce the excessive turnover of psoriatic epidermal cells. All antimetabolites have significant side effects and require careful monitoring. Methotrexate is the drug best studied and most commonly used. Antimetabolites are best left to the experts; anyone attempting their use should carefully review the recent literature.

Corticosteroids

Systemic corticosteroids are rarely indicated in the treatment of psoriasis. Psoriatic erythroderma may be one exception. Although systemic corticosteroids are temporarily dramatically effective in controlling psoriasis, the disease flares up severely when side effects require their withdrawal. Few things are more difficult than weaning a psoriatic patient from long-term corticosteroids.

Psoralens

The use of psoralens plus ultraviolet light—photochemotherapy—is mentioned under the section on ultraviolet light therapy.

Etretinate

Etretinate, a new vitamin A derivative, is effective in suppressing the severer forms of psoriasis. It has not yet been approved and its safety for long-term treatment is unknown.

X-ray therapy

Superficial X-ray and grenz-ray therapy is often effective in suppressing psoriasis. Many dermatologists use it successfully to provide temporary clearing of stubborn, localized psoriasis. As a therapeutic tool in psoriasis, X-ray therapy is of limited value. Psoriasis is a chronic, usually lifetime disease, yet the total amount of X-ray exposure that may be given is limited.

Managing the patient

Psoriasis presents a challenge in psychological management as much as in clinical therapy. Psoriasis is not psychosomatic; part of the psychological management of psoriasis is to stress that psoriasis is not caused by nerves or emotions but is a genetically determined defect of skin growth. It's bad enough to have psoriasis; the patient shouldn't have to feel guilty about being responsible for it. This is not to deny that emotional stress may aggravate psoriasis, just as it does many other somatic disorders.

The emotional impact of psoriasis is often overwhelming. The advertisements referring to the "heartbreak of psoriasis" don't exaggerate its effects on some patients. The true physician prescribes more than topical medicaments; he helps and supports patients' efforts to cope with this disorder. The patient must understand the course of psoriasis and the limitations of treatment. Explain that treatment will be a long haul and that there is no magical cure. It helps to point out that this is also true for diabetes, hypertension, and arthritis.

It's equally important to reassure patients with stable, chronic psoriasis of a few areas (e.g., scalp, elbows, perianal area) that in all likelihood their psoriasis will remain a localized nuisance. Only a small percentage of psoriatics have severe, "life-ruining" eruptions.

Approach treatment with enthusiasm and provide specific instructions so that the patient realizes you have a therapeutic program in mind and aren't groping in the dark. Avoid the "You might try this ointment" approach. Remind discouraged patients that psoriasis often improves spontaneously and may clear up for many years.

31

Rosacea

Etiology

Rosacea is a skin dysfunction characterized by papulopustules and areas of erythema. Its resemblance to acne is emphasized by the antiquated term for this disorder, acne rosacea. Its cause is unknown. Older textbooks often discuss fancied relationships to emotions, diets, and/or gastrointestinal disorders. Eye disorders—chiefly conjunctivitis, rarely keratitis—occasionally accompany rosacea.

Diagnosis

Diagnosis is easy in the *typical* case with both papulopustules and areas of erythema. Unlike acne vulgaris, the nose is usually prominently affected (Figure C-38). Sometimes, when papulopustules are sparse, seborrheic dermatitis, discoid LE, and eczema enter into the differential diagnosis. The chronic application of fluorinated corticosteroids to the skin of the face can produce a dermatitis closely resembling rosacea, which has been termed "rosacea-like dermatitis from steroids," "steroid rosacea," and "corticosteroid facies." Atypical forms of rosacea are common and often not recognized.

Treatment

Systemic antibiotics, especially tetracyclines, are usually dramatically effective in suppressing the papulopustules of rosacea (Figures C-39, C-40, and C-41). The effect of antibiotics on the erythema of rosacea is less marked and often disappointing. Antibiotics only suppress rosacea and do not change its chronic, relapsing course. Once rosacea is established, long-term treatment is usually necessary. While some patients require tetracycline for years, others are able to decrease their antibiotic gradually and, after several months, stop it. However, even those fortunate enough to be able to stop their antibiotics should be warned that a recurrence is likely within the next year or two—and that the course of rosacea is unpredictable. Long-term antibiotic suppression of rosacea is important when there is severe nose involvement, since uncontrolled rosacea of the nose may lead to rhinophyma (Figure C-38). Similarly, significant eye symptoms are an indication for continuing antibiotic suppression.

Tetracycline is the most widely used antibiotic in rosacea. Doses as low as 250 or 500 mg a day are often effective. My preference is to start with the conventional adult dose of 1 gm a day for one month. It's logical to determine first whether or not tetracycline will be effective, and later to find the smallest dose necessary. If 1 gm of tetracycline is effective in suppressing rosacea, the patient gradually reduces the dose by 250 mg at a time at four- to six-week intervals; this is similar to the approach suggested for acne. In general, rosacea responds both more rapidly and more readily to tetracycline than does acne. As an aid to the systematic decrease of tetracycline, use the long-term tetracycline instruction sheet.

If the patient fails to improve on 1 gm of tetracycline per day, I usually employ a trial of erythromycin, 1 gm a day. When there is a partial response to 1 gm of tetracycline a day, increase the tetracycline to 1.5 gm a day. Such an increase is usually well tolerated, except that in sunny climes phototoxicity may prove a problem. Whatever the antibiotic and dose used, once a satisfactory response has been obtained, the patient gradually reduces the dose to find the smallest maintenance dose that will control his rosacea.

What to do for the patient who dislikes taking, or does not tolerate, systemic antibiotics? Topical formulations used for acne (see Chapter 4) may provide some control. While the traditional treatment of rosacea includes topicals containing tar or sulfur, they're probably ineffective. Fluorinated corticosteroid topicals should not be used, as they may aggravate or cause rosacea (Figure C-39).

32

Scabies

Etiology

Scabies results from infestation with the mite *Sarcoptes scabiei*. Scabies is a fascinating disorder that occurs in periodic epidemics and then almost vanishes from the medical scene.

Diagnosis

Diagnosis depends on the physician's index of suspicion and experience. While typical cases can be diagnosed at a glance by the experienced, scabies can present in unusual fashions that fool even the experts. Suspect scabies when dealing with any intensely itching eruption that spares the face. The review by Orkin and Maibach is brief, excellent, and current.[1]

The diagnosis of scabies can be proven by demonstrating the mite, a challenging task. Although a patient with scabies may have hundreds of itching papules, he often has fewer than a dozen mites. The generalized eruption (Figure C-42) is a hypersensitivity response. Your chances of finding a typical burrow and extracting a mite are best on the hands and wrists, especially the webs between fingers (Figure C-43). Sometimes the ankles yield burrows; in males the penis should be carefully examined. The burrow is a short line that resembles a superficial scratch except that it's curved or wavy (Figures C-44 and C-45). The tiny blackish dot at one end is the mite. A magnifying glass or binocular loupe is almost essential in the search.

When you've located a suspected burrow, you can confirm the mite's presence microscopically in either of two ways:

1. If you see a tiny black dot at one end, this is probably the mite; insert a small hypodermic needle (25- or 26-gauge) or the tip of a pointed scalpel blade into the skin. The mite will stick to it and can be transferred to some glycerol, water, or immersion oil on a slide, covered with a coverslip, and examined under low power. Extracting the mite with a needle is the best way, but requires experience.

2. An alternative approach is to slice off the whole burrow with a sterile

scalpel blade held parallel to the skin. You will draw some blood if you do this properly. Put the slice on a slide, cover it with glycerol or mineral or immersion oil, add a coverslip, and examine it under a microscope. The presence of the mite, ova, or feces—small, brownish, rounded objects—proves the diagnosis. When you can't find any burrows, try vigorously scraping an area of multiple papules or excoriations in the finger webs or wrists and examining the scrapings after clearing with one of the above media.

Even the most expert will sometimes fail to prove the diagnosis. If there are strong clinical suspicions of scabies, a therapeutic trial is indicated even if the mite can't be demonstrated. A therapeutic trial should be just that: a one- or possibly two-time application of a scabicide.

Contagion

Scabies is cured by killing the mite. The patient will stay cured only if the possibility of reinfection is eliminated. This means treatment of close contacts. There are many misconceptions about the contagiousness of scabies; it requires *close personal contact*. In our society, transmission between adults is usually the result of sexual activity. Child-to-child and child-to-adult transfer occurs readily without sex. Scabies is practically never spread by clothing or bedding. There's no need to call in exterminators or process bedding or clothing in any special manner. By 24 hours after effective treatment, scabies is no longer contagious.

How wide to spread the treatment net in an effort to eradicate all potential sources of the mite remains controversial. Some physicians treat only those contacts they have personally examined and found to harbor scabies. I believe this approach impractical, not only because it may be virtually impossible to get all contacts in for a medical examination but also because early scabies may be overlooked even by a skilled examiner. I believe it best to treat *all* sexual contacts and all family members of a patient with proven scabies. *Proven* usually means that the mite has been demonstrated, although when two or more members of a family—or sexual partners—have a clinical picture typical of scabies there's little likelihood of anything else.

Treatment

There are no data as to which scabicide is best. Currently 1 per cent gamma benzene hexachloride (Kwell) lotion or cream is most popular in North America. It is effective and only moderately irritating. Its drawback is neurotoxicity, which has been a problem clinically only when it has been greatly overused in small children. However, many physicians prefer not to use it in small children or pregnant women. Crotamiton (Eurax) cream is an alternative that's apparently relatively nontoxic. Benzyl benzoate is a very effective scabicide, available only with difficulty in North America and therefore not widely used by United States physicians. Sulfur ointment (5 per cent)—a centuries-old remedy—is little used now except when there's concern about the toxicity of gamma benzene hexachloride. Benzyl benzoate and sulfur preparations are irritating and tend to produce dermatitis.

The currently recommended treatment regimen is a single evening application of 1 per cent gamma benzene hexachloride lotion to the entire body from the neck downward. The medication is to be thoroughly rubbed into the hands and wrists and the hands not washed. The patient bathes 24 hours later. For pregnant women and children under the age of 2 years, crotamiton ointment is used instead, being applied at bedtime for two nights in a row to the entire body from the neck down. It's important that all family members and sexual partners be treated on the same night.

While the official recommendation is for just one application of gamma benzene hexachloride, many experienced clinicians use two applications spaced one week apart. The two-application approach may be indicated in those with a varied sexual life to catch any Ping-Pong reinfection from sexual partners not treated at the same time.

These schedules are provided with the caveat that they are not the optimal treatment—no one knows the best treatment for scabies. The methods described work for the majority of patients and appear safe. It's important that when gamma benzene hexachloride is used, two applications at the most be employed. Prescriptions should be nonrefillable and patients specifically warned not to apply it more than once (or twice if you so order). To prevent overtreatment, prescribe only enough scabicide for treatment of the patient and contacts: 30 ml of cream or lotion suffice for one application per adult.

In my practice, accompanying dermatitis is so common that virtually all adult patients are also given a 10- to 14-day tapering course of prednisone by mouth. When there are signs of secondary infection with oozing and crusts, a five- to seven-day course of an oral antibiotic such as erythromycin is indicated in addition.

I routinely tell patients with dermatitis to avoid soap and to use bath oils or other lubricants if their skin is too dry. Generally patients are requested to return in two weeks, since postscabetic dermatitis is quite common. Postscabetic dermatitis usually yields to a two- to three-week tapering course of prednisone combined with topical corticosteroids and avoidance of soap. Occasionally longer courses of systemic corticosteroids are necessary. When this happens, try to shift the patient to every-other-day prednisone taken as a single dose in the morning. The follow-up examination reassures the patient that any continuing itching is not due to scabies. This lessens the temptation for patients to reuse their scabicide whenever they itch—which patients do in spite of strict warnings to the contrary.

Complications

Postscabetic dermatitis is the main problem and occasionally goes on for months, with persistent itching nodules. Men may develop indurated, severely itching scrotal and inguinal nodules. When it's impossible to distinguish postscabetic dermatitis from a treatment failure, a second course of antiscabetic therapy is permitted. Unfortunately, not infrequently patients use potent antiscabetic agents daily for weeks and even months with the mistaken notion that their persistent itching represents persistent scabies. Therefore, do not make your prescriptions for scabicides refillable.

Reference

1. Orkin M, Maibach HI: This scabies pandemic. *N Engl J Med* 289:496, 1978

Seborrheic keratoses

33

Etiology

Seborrheic keratoses are benign, genetically determined growths that usually appear first in adulthood. They gradually increase in number. Elderly patients may have a great many keratoses covering the trunk (see Figure C-16). They are not caused by sun damage. Their former name of seborrheic verruca is appropriate to these wartlike lesions.

Diagnosis

Differential diagnosis includes viral warts, nevi, actinic keratoses, basal-cell carcinoma, squamous-cell carcinoma, and, when the keratoses are highly pigmented, malignant melanoma.

Treatment

There are two indications for treatment: (1) The diagnosis is in question and/or (2) the patient wants the growths removed. Seborrheic keratoses may itch, are often unsightly, or may otherwise be annoying to the patient.

The superficial nature of seborrheic keratoses makes removal easy by either curettage or liquid nitrogen freezing. If there's a question of diagnosis, curette them to provide a specimen for histology. Otherwise the choice between liquid nitrogen and curettage depends on the availability of liquid nitrogen and your preference.

While cosmetic results with liquid nitrogen are slightly superior to those obtained by curettage, on the face either method produces excellent results—often without any scars. In treating seborrheic keratoses of the trunk and extremities, both curettage and liquid nitrogen frequently leave slight scars. Liquid nitrogen may produce temporary hyperpigmentation. The slight scarring that either method may cause is much preferable to the appearance of the original growths.

Liquid nitrogen technique is discussed in Chapter 3. Judging the depth of adequate liquid nitrogen freezing can be difficult. I tend to be conservative

143

and freeze seborrheic keratoses lightly. The patient is asked to return for a no-charge checkup visit in four to five weeks and is told that any residual keratoses will be frozen a second time without additional charge. Remember that you can always freeze a second time—but the scar from too heavy-handed a use of liquid nitrogen can never be undone.

Removal by curettage is simple. After giving local anesthesia, stretch the skin with the fingers of one hand and, using a 5- or 6-mm-diameter curette, scrape off the keratoses to a clean base with short, firm strokes. If optimum cosmetic results are critical, use pressure or gelatin foam to control bleeding. Otherwise you can use a styptic such as Monsel's solution. Do not electrodesiccate keratoses, as that needlessly increases scarring. Details of curettage treatment and aftercare are discussed in the unit on postoperative care.

Seborrheic keratoses

Skin aging and solar damage

34

In our youth-oriented society, skin aging is a frequent concern of patients. Much of what is commonly referred to as skin aging—fine wrinkles, irregular pigmentation, and patchy roughness—is not the result of age but a consequence of sun damage. Fair-skinned persons are especially prone to such effects; darker-skinned persons suffer less sun damage, thanks to the protection provided by their pigment. It's common to underestimate the age of middle-aged blacks, since their youthful-appearing skin represents an absence of actinic damage. Not all skin "aging" is caused by sun damage; age is responsible for the deep wrinkles of the elderly.

The deleterious effects of sun damage are not fully appreciated. We've forgotten the wisdom of our great-grandmothers, who, with wide-brimmed hats, gloves, long sleeves, and parasols, carefully avoided the sun. Not only does sunlight age skin, but it's also responsible for basal-cell carcinomas (which hardly ever occur in blacks) and most squamous-cell carcinomas. Sunlight plays a role in the etiology of malignant melanoma. It's suspected that the increasing incidence of malignant melanoma—a worldwide phenomenon—is related to the sun worship so widely practiced. The idea of preventing disease has become fashionable; we can help prevent disease caused by the sun.

As in other forms of radiation injury, there is a latent interval between sun exposure and the appearance of skin damage. Youthful sunbathing is a time bomb that may not go off for decades. Sun damage is cumulative and irreversible. A common misconception is that sun damage is caused by sunburn and that moderate sun exposure is safe. Not true; moderate sun exposure and careful tanning will avoid sunburn but not actinic damage. Actinic damage is permanent, since we can't rejuvenate the skin.

A widespread misconception—encouraged by cosmetics manufacturers—is that systematic (or "regular") skin lubrication and use of moisturizers prevent wrinkling and skin aging. Skin lubricants, moisturizers, and similar preparations frequently make skin appear smoother and more appealing for a few hours after use; however, they confer no permanent benefit. Tell patients that moisturizers and skin lotions provide only a temporary lubricating effect. Furthermore, reassure them that soap and water will not permanently dry and wrinkle their skin. Minimizing sun exposure is the only way to stave off the stigmata of aging skin.

Solar damage is produced by the sunlight's invisible ultraviolet rays. Clothing provides the best protection from these rays; sunscreens should be used on uncovered parts of the body. The most effective sunscreens contain pigment and mechanically block sunlight. The paint-like pigments make them unsightly and messy. Nevertheless, they are effective and practical when appearance is not at a premium; note the widespread use of zinc oxide to protect nose and lips at the beach. Commercial preparations of this type (A-Fil ointment, RVPaque ointment) are given a flesh-colored tint to make them cosmetically more acceptable. A thick, heavily colored makeup base is also an efficient sun protective.

Most sun protectives are "clean," transparent preparations that act by chemically absorbing ultraviolet rays. The best ultraviolet absorbers are PABA (*p*-aminobenzoic acid) or its derivatives and the benzophenones. Some PABA formulations are adsorbed to a moderate degree on the stratum corneum, resist washing, and provide some sunlight protection during swimming if applied one or two hours beforehand. Allergy to PABA and its derivatives occurs occasionally; PABA is chemically related to benzocaine. Instruct patients to try PABA-containing sun protectives on a small area of skin for several days to see if they are tolerated.

The sun-protective factor is a quantitative measure of a sunscreen's efficacy. It's the ratio of the amount of light needed to produce erythema in the presence of a sunscreen to the amount of light producing erythema with no sunscreen. The higher the number, the better the protection. Patients should use a product with an SPF of 15, currently the highest meaningful ratio.

There are many efficient over-the-counter sun protectives containing PABA, a PABA derivative, or a benzophenone, sometimes in combination. I won't even try to list the many and changing brand names. The patient instruction sheet has blank spaces for names to be inserted; you may wish to provide samples as well as specific brand names.

Patients frequently ask, "Will I tan when using a sun blocker?" "Unfortunately, yes," is the answer. Even the most efficient clean sun protectives allow a significant amount of solar radiation to reach the skin. Tell patients they should try to prevent tanning, for it's impossible to tan without the skin undergoing damage.

Lips should be protected from the sun with an ultraviolet-absorbing lip pomade (sunStick, RVPaba lipstick) or a heavily pigmented lipstick. Ordinary lubricating lip pomades do not give adequate protection.

Body lotions, baby oil, and tanning creams are frequently used by sunbathers who believe these preparations afford significant sun protection. They do not. Tanning lotions are simply weak sun protectors designed to screen out some of the ultraviolet light to minimize the risk of a sunburn.

Detailed advice regarding sun protection is given in the patient instruction sheet. Patients will appreciate your specific recommendations of sun protectives. Tell your patients that expensive moisturizers, creams, and lubricants won't prevent wrinkles and skin aging. If they like the feel of a skin lubricant, suggest they buy an inexpensive brand. Emphasize that systematic use of sun-protective measures will prevent premature wrinkles.

Aim at moderation. The message is to minimize sun exposure, not avoid it. Occasionally one encounters patients who have become so frightened of sun exposure that they've renounced all outdoor activities. Such overreaction is rare; it's more common for patients to continue their avid sun worship in spite of our warnings.

Tetracycline treatment of acneiform disorders

35

Acne, rosacea, and rosaceaform disorders (perioral dermatitis) often require long-term tetracycline therapy for suppression. About 90 per cent of patients with rosacea or perioral dermatitis do well with tetracycline suppression (see Figures C-39, C-40, and C-41). With acne the response is less certain; probably fewer than two-thirds of acne cases respond satisfactorily to the usual doses of tetracycline. Rosacea and acne are long-term disorders that may require years of antibiotic suppression. Most perioral dermatitis clears up in a matter of months, although sometimes it too takes a long, dragged-out course. Since topical therapy offers little benefit to these patients, long-term control means long-term ingestion of antibiotics, usually tetracycline.

The long-term use of systemic antibiotics to treat what are essentially cosmetically handicapping skin disorders runs counter to traditional medical teaching. Haven't we all been told to use antibiotics sparingly, and only for definitely diagnosed bacterial infections? Yet nearly all dermatologists—and many other physicians as well—prescribe enormous amounts of tetracycline in treating acne, rosacea, and perioral dermatitis. Patients frequently voice concern about the long-term effect of tetracycline.

Fortunately, there's good evidence that long-term tetracycline therapy is remarkably safe. Several careful studies, as well as extensive clinical experience, have shown that patients on long-term tetracycline therapy are just as healthy as those who aren't. There's no need to monitor tetracycline therapy with blood counts and urinalyses.

Women taking tetracycline should be told to stop it if they become pregnant. Tetracycline is apparently not teratogenic; however, it's incorporated into the fetal bones and teeth, and this is not desirable. Gastrointestinal distress and yeast vaginitis—fairly common side effects of tetracycline—usually appear early and so are seldom problems in long-term therapy.

Photosensitivity is a troubling side effect in sunnier climes. Photosensitivity is dose-related and is rarely a problem when the daily dosage of tetracycline is 500 mg or less. With 1 gm daily most fair-skinned persons will observe easier sunburning when exposed to summer sunshine. Individuals taking 2 gm of tetracycline a day invariably experience easy sunburning.

148

Photo-onycholysis—separation of the nails from their bases as a result of sun exposure—is an occasional side effect, mainly in young women taking 1 gm or more of tetracycline daily. For some reason, photo-onycholysis occurs more commonly in women than in men. While tetracycline photosensitivity in North American patients is a problem principally during summer, be sure to alert skiers and patients taking a midwinter vacation on a sunny island. The patient information sheet warns about sun sensitivity and advises the use of sun-protective measures. You may wish to hand those patients on higher doses of tetracycline—or who are heavily exposed to the sun—the patient instruction sheet "Sunlight and Your Skin."

The patient instructions stress the safety of long-term tetracycline treatment. Be sure to mention this to patients. It will not only help to reassure them but also open the way for them to voice their concerns and fears. Not infrequently patients have heard that it's dangerous to take antibiotics for a long time. An occasional patient worries about addiction. Stress that tetracycline has no mood-altering effects.

In long-term tetracycline therapy, the aim is to take the minimum dose required to suppress the eruption effectively. Since this minimum effective dose can vary widely, it needs to be determined for each person. After you've determined that full doses of tetracycline are effective, the next step is to reduce the dose gradually to the point of a mild flare-up to determine the smallest amount required.

The patient instruction sheet provides a schedule with dates and number of tablets to be filled in by the physician. Since there's a significant lag between taking tetracycline and the appearance of its effect, decreases in tetracycline dose should be gradual. Generally four to six weeks should be allowed at one dose level before further reduction is attempted. Stress that patients should follow their schedules and reduce their tetracycline only gradually.

With some guidance, most patients adjust their tetracycline dosages successfully. Patients are told that they may adjust their dosages upward to the previous original amounts if pimples break out on lower doses. This is especially important to those patients whose acne is improved with summer sunshine but flares up during fall and winter. Occasionally a patient varies the dosage from day to day, depending on how many pimples he finds in the morning. This practice should be stopped and the reason why it's pointless explained. Once patients understand that there is a lag of one to three weeks between the ingestion of tetracycline and the appearance of its effect, they recognize the uselessness of day-to-day adjustments.

Tetracycline should be taken on an empty stomach, since food, especially dairy products, binds it in the gastrointestinal tract and interferes with absorption. Taking tetracycline split into two daily doses is as effective as—and simpler than—the older, four-times-a-day regimen. A simple system will help your patients remember to take their antibiotic regularly. Tell the patient to count out the entire day's antibiotic ration when entering the bathroom upon arising. Stress that this should be done even before using the toilet. The patient should take one half of the daily tetracycline ration at once with a full glass of water and put the other half in a small glass bottle or dish in a prominent place in the bathroom (assuming there are no small children about). The container with the medication serves as a reminder for the patient to take it in the evening. Ask the patient to check the dish at bedtime; and if it isn't empty, he's to take his dose then, as he obviously forgot it earlier. When a patient is taking two tablets or less of tetracycline daily, the entire dose is taken at one time on arising. This simple routine virtually eliminates forgotten doses—not an uncommon problem with patients on long-term oral therapy.

How frequently should you ask patients on long-term tetracycline therapy to return? In general, acne patients require closer follow-up than patients with rosacea. Rosacea tends to run a more stable course than acne, and one is dealing with adults, who are more reliable than adolescents about taking long-term medications. It would seem wise to see acne patients taking long-term tetracycline therapy every three months for the first half year and then, if their skin eruptions are reasonably well controlled on relatively small (i.e., less than 1-gm) doses of tetracycline daily, see them every six months to one year thereafter. Patients should be told that if their acne is not adequately controlled, they should return promptly. There's no point in taking any medicine if it's ineffective.

Tinea cruris ("jock itch")

36

Etiology

Tinea cruris is an infection of the skin of the groin with fungi, notably *Trichophyton mentagrophytes*, *Trichophyton rubrum*, and *Epidermophyton floccosum*. Tinea cruris is frequent in males, rare in women. "Jock itch" is a lay term referring to any itchy groin rash.

Diagnosis

Tinea cruris usually shows sharply demarcated, scaling patches (the old term was eczema marginatum) extending from the inguinal folds onto the thighs and often the buttocks. A fine collarette of scales or tiny papules is often present. Finding typical hyphae on microscopy of KOH-cleared skin scrapings taken from the edge of the lesion clinches the diagnosis. Candidiasis, nonspecific intertrigo, seborrheic dermatitis, and psoriasis are the chief differential diagnostic problems (see Figure C-37).

It used to be important to distinguish candidiasis from tinea cruris, since the treatments of these disorders differed. Fortunately, there are now effective topical fungicides that act against both tinea cruris and candidiasis. Most traditional fungicides are ineffective against yeasts, and anti-*Candida* agents such as nystatin (Mycostatin, Nilstat) and amphotericin (Fungizone) are not effective against the dermatophytes causing tinea cruris. It isn't uncommon to encounter patients who have been unsuccessfully treating their tinea cruris with a nystatin preparation prescribed by a physician who mistakenly thought the preparation was antifungal.

Candidiasis usually shows satellite lesions beyond the border of the main rash, and superficial vesicles that may have ruptured, leaving small, round, denuded areas. Seborrheic dermatitis of the groin and inguinal psoriasis can perfectly mimic tinea cruris. It isn't rare to have tinea cruris coexist with groin psoriasis; here confirmation of the diagnosis by microscopy of skin scrapings is essential.

A frequent complication is superimposed dermatitis from excessive scrubbing with soap and water or application of irritating remedies. The dermatitis can mislead the physician by obscuring the underlying tinea cruris. The inguinal folds are particularly prone to irritation from topical medicaments. This often leads to a remarkable similarity in appearance of groin rashes of different etiologies.

Treatment

General principles

Tinea cruris usually responds promptly to the newer topical broad-spectrum fungicides. Unfortunately, recurrences are common, especially when the infecting organism is *T. rubrum*. Dermatophytes thrive in a moist, warm environment; flare-ups and recurrences of tinea cruris are likely during hot weather, after prolonged wearing of a bathing suit, and with heavy sweating. Patients with persistent or recurrent tinea cruris should be advised to wear loose cotton underwear and use a bland dusting powder in the groin. Prophylactic use of tolnaftate powder sometimes works wonders; it's an over-the-counter fungicide (Tinactin) that's well tolerated in the groin.

When dermatitis coexists with tinea cruris, the two disorders must be treated simultaneously. The combined use of a corticosteroid topical and antifungal topical is wise. Depending on severity, you may combine a brief course of oral prednisone with topical antifungals or prescribe griseofulvin by mouth and a topical corticosteroid. Prescribe only gentle measures. Topicals that itch, burn, or aggravate the eruption should be stopped.

Groin skin is easily irritated. Instruct patients not to apply home remedies. Soap should not be used on the groin; cleansing with plain water suffices. Soap may be used on normal skin when showering, since transient contact with dilute soapy water does no harm.

Specific treatment

Systemic
Griseofulvin (Fulvicin, Grifulvin, Grisactin) promptly clears tinea cruris. It should be reserved for severe cases that don't respond to topical fungicides. Not only may systemic griseofulvin produce significant side effects, but it's a carcinogen in mice and is being used with increasing reluctance in humans. However, its occasional use is justified, especially when tinea cruris coexists with another skin disorder such as psoriasis.

Topical
The newer broad-spectrum fungicides—miconazole (Monistat), clotrimazole (Lotrimin, Mycelex), and haloprogin (Halotex)—are best. My current favorites are clotrimazole cream and miconazole cream. They have the advantage of also being anti-*Candida* agents and are less irritating than older preparations containing undecylenic acid. However, even these broad-spectrum fungicides are moderately irritating and should be used sparingly. In the groin, the cream formulations are better tolerated than liquids. Iodochlorhydroxy-

quin (Vioform) is a less effective fungicide and has the drawback of staining clothes. I consider it obsolete, although some physicians are fond of it.

While simple, uncomplicated tinea cruris usually responds to topical fungicides, this is not the case when there's accompanying dermatitis. When tinea cruris and dermatitis coexist, treatment with a topical corticosteroid-fungicide combination is frequently effective. In the United States, unfortunately, the only commercial corticosteroid-fungicide combination is iodochlorhydroxyquin-hydrocortisone (Vioform-Hydrocortisone), which I consider obsolete because of its weak antifungal action. Pharmacists can readily add 1 to 2 per cent hydrocortisone powder to miconazole or clotrimazole cream to make an effective, nonstaining (albeit expensive) combination. Another approach is to alternate a fungicide with 2 to 3 per cent hydrocortisone cream, applying each two or three times a day. Fluorinated corticosteroids are best avoided in the groin; they tend to cause atrophy and striae.

When there is severe dermatitis, avoid topical fungicides. Because the inflammatory process causes shedding of the fungi, fungicides are usually unnecessary in this stage and are likely to irritate the already inflamed skin. Once the acute dermatitis has been controlled, fungicides—either alone or in combination with hydrocortisone—are often beneficial.

37

Tinea versicolor

Etiology

Tinea versicolor is a superficial fungal infection caused by *Malassezia furfur*, which is identical with the microorganism *Pityrosporon orbiculare* found on normal skin. Tinea versicolor is caused by overgrowth of an inhabitant of normal skin. It is not contagious.

Patients usually seek treatment because their lesions are cosmetically annoying; rarely there is slight itching. Tinea versicolor is more common in the tropics and often flares up in hot weather.

Diagnosis

Tinea versicolor is characterized by variable coloring and mild scaling. Patches of tinea versicolor are lighter than tanned skin and often give the impression of vitiligo. Occasionally tinea versicolor is misdiagnosed as vitiligo. Close examination, however, shows fine scaling—absent in vitiligo— and usually tinea versicolor shows only partial pigment loss. On untanned skin the patches of tinea versicolor are pinkish to coppery and are darker than the surrounding skin. Seborrheic dermatitis, pityriasis rosea, and sometimes tinea corporis are the chief differential diagnoses.

Microscopy of KOH-cleared scrapings, a useful diagnostic tool, shows short, curved hyphae and clusters of round yeast cells. Examination of the skin under ultraviolet black light (Wood's light) may be helpful, in that active lesions may have a yellowish fluorescence. This is often absent, however, and black-light examination is less useful as a diagnostic aid than to demonstrate the extent of the process—which is usually more widespread than ordinary light reveals.

Treatment

Many remedies clear up this disorder, but clearing is usually temporary since the disease is not the result of infection by an exogenous agent, but overgrowth of a normal skin inhabitant. Sooner or later tinea versicolor recurs. Not only do we lack a cure, we don't even know which of the many recommended treatments is best.

It's difficult to know when to stop treatment if depigmentation is prominent. Treatment does not repigment the skin; once tinea versicolor has cleared up, the skin will repigment normally. Prescribe a course of treatment, and wait one or two months for the color contrast to fade. If the color contrast persists or scaling continues, repeat the treatment.

Many dermatologists use 2.5 per cent selenium sulfide suspension dandruff shampoo (Selsun, Exsel). The method I use is a single, thorough application of selenium sulfide suspension at bedtime, removed by showering in the morning. Some physicians advise repeating the overnight application once weekly for a month. I treat just once, wait one month, and then repeat the overnight treatment if the patient's skin isn't clear. An alternative selenium sulfide regimen is to apply the suspension once daily for four consecutive days; keep it on for 30 minutes each time, and wash the medicine off thoroughly in the shower at the end of each treatment. Selenium sulfide is cheap and usually effective.

If selenium sulfide fails—or when a different treatment is desired—a salicylic acid-containing "peeling" medicament applied sparingly at bedtime is frequently effective. Examples of such preparations are 3 to 5 per cent salicylic acid in isopropyl alcohol (readily prepared by a pharmacist), Whitfield's ointment (cheap but messy), or a commercial salicylic acid-containing gel (Saligel, over-the-counter). Nightly applications of 50 per cent propylene glycol in water are often effective. This preparation is both cheap and clean. The newer antifungal agents such as miconazole (Monistat), clotrimazole (Lotrimin, Mycelex), and haloprogin (Halotex) are effective in treating tinea versicolor, but they're expensive and no more effective than the less-expensive medications discussed above. Sodium thiosulfate, a traditional remedy, stinks and requires numerous applications; use something else.

Tinea versicolor recurs almost routinely. Tell your patients to repeat the treatment when—not if—tinea versicolor recurs. Prophylactic treatment is one way of dealing with recurrences; a single overnight application of selenium sulfide every three months is effective.

38

Warts

Diagnosis

Diagnosis of warts is usually easy; most patients make the correct diagnosis themselves. An exception is plantar warts, which may closely resemble corns. Often it's necessary to pare down a plantar callus before the characteristic speckled appearance of the plantar wart is evident. Lesions of molluscum contagiosum may resemble warts until, on closer inspection, molluscum contagiosum's smooth papule with umbilication is recognized. Warts always have a rough surface. At times warts may be indistinguishable from seborrheic keratoses. Flat warts can closely resemble benign keratoses or epidermal nevi; when grouped, they're sometimes mistaken for a rash.

Treatment

General principles

Does anyone enjoy treating warts? Warts appear to have a bad reputation among primary physicians, since warty patients are frequently referred to dermatologists for "expert" therapy. Yet the unpredictable nature of warts "ruins dermatologists' reputations," as one dermatologist puts it.

Since there are no systemic antiwart viral agents, *unsatisfactory* best describes the destructive methods we employ. Warts often fail to disappear with treatment, or they recur after apparent cure. Fortunately nature helps, as warts may disappear by themselves, especially in children. This tendency of warts to disappear spontaneously makes it difficult to evaluate treatments. There is no way of preventing warts, and both patient and physician may become discouraged by an apparently endless succession of new warts.

The goal of treatment is to destroy the wart while sparing normal skin. Many people have scars from overenthusiastic wart destruction—often by electrodesiccation. Scars on the face or legs are unsightly; on the soles they may be painful. Warts do not produce scars; scars are the result of treatment.

The benign nature of warts requires that treatment be limited to methods that have proven safe. This excludes—with rare exceptions—X-ray therapy.

Deliberately sensitizing patients to a potent allergen such as dinitrochlorobenzene, followed by application of the sensitizer to warts to produce a brisk dermatitis, is an experimental procedure. I don't recommend it. The same warnings apply to the use of live vaccines to inoculate warts. Be skeptical of "new" wart treatments; few are effective, and some are dangerous.

The absence of a truly effective wart treatment makes it important that the patient understand that warts are unpredictable. This book includes a background information sheet on warts that's suitable for all warty patients. Once adequately informed, patients will—I hope—blame treatment failures or the development of new warts on the capricious wart virus rather than on your treatment.

A great variety of thermal and chemical irritants have been proclaimed effective in treating warts. Repeated irritation of the wart is the common factor in these remedies. It's speculated that repeated irritation alters the body's response to warts, probably by some immune process, and causes wart necrosis. No one agent is superior, in this respect, since the actions of these irritants are nonspecific.

Most dermatologists have simple wart treatment routines. The trick is that different types of warts require different routines. You must tailor the treatment to the wart's structure and location. From the standpoint of treatment warts can be grouped into (1) verruca vulgaris, the common wart; (2) plantar warts, warts of the sole; (3) flat warts; (4) acuminate (moist) warts on the mucocutaneous junctions of the anogenital area; and (5) periungual warts.

Specific step-by-step directions for treating each type of wart are given in the next section. Look upon those detailed directions as a collection of wart treatment recipes; review and follow them just as a cook carefully follows a new recipe. The instructions are designed so that the occasional wart therapist can proceed with confidence. As repetition brings familiarity, you'll find yourself referring to them less and less frequently.

Before scanning the specifics of wart treatment, please carefully read the remainder of this section on general principles. An understanding of why certain methods are advisable—and why others are not—will help you avoid unpleasant results and unhappy patients.

At times a wart persists no matter what you do. If tissue histology confirms the diagnosis of wart (carcinoma can masquerade as warts), advise the patient to live with the wart. Suggesting that the wart may disappear spontaneously (as it may) helps the patient tolerate it.

Here's a true story: I struggled unsuccessfully with a persistent wart on the third toe of a 62-year-old woman. The wart resisted chemical destruction, repeated liquid nitrogen treatments, and two curette removals. Histology confirmed the diagnosis. I suggested that the patient live with her wart and pare it down when it became protuberant. Unwilling to accept this, she sought treatment from another dermatologist, who included a course of X-ray therapy along with many other unsuccessful remedies. Subsequent excision and grafting by a plastic surgeon failed to eradicate the tenacious growth. Later, while hospitalized for a cholecystectomy, the woman persuaded an orthopedic surgeon to amputate her toe! This got rid of the wart, of course, but left her with persistent pain at the amputation site. Fortunately, such horror stories are rare.

Specific methods

This section provides detailed instructions for treating the five types of warts. The methods are practical and safe. Some warts are best treated at home by chemical destruction. To be successful, these self-treatment approaches require careful instruction of patients. This will be made easier by using the patient instruction sheets titled "Chemical Destruction of Warts" and "Plantar Warts."

Verruca vulgaris (common wart)

Surgery

Surgical treatment of the common wart is rapidly and easily accomplished by scoop removal, using scissors and curette, and has a better than 90 per cent cure rate. This simple surgical method usually results in a small, sometimes invisible scar. Because even a tiny scar on the sole can be troublesome, surgery should be avoided in treating plantar warts. In cosmetically significant areas such as the face, elbows, and knees, liquid nitrogen treatment is preferable, although gentle scissors and curette removal usually provides cosmetically acceptable results if only pressure or gelatin foam packing is used for hemostasis.

Surgical treatment of warts by scoop removal or blunt dissection is described in detail in Chapter 3. Following local anesthesia, the epidermis is incised circumferentially around the wart with the tip of a small, curved scissors. Using a large curette or a blunt dissector, a cleavage plane is established around the wart, and the wart is shelled out. Bleeding is controlled by applying Monsel's solution or, if you are very concerned about scarring, by pressure or packing with gelatin foam. Electrodesiccation should be avoided in treating ordinary warts, for it unnecessarily increases scarring. Surgical wart removal means scissors and curette removal—never full-scale excision and suture. Since warts are neoplasms limited to the epidermis, full-thickness skin excision is overdoing things.

Liquid nitrogen treatment

From a cosmetic viewpoint, liquid nitrogen is an excellent treatment for warts. It's the treatment of choice for warts of the face and cosmetically sensitive areas of the hands, arms, and legs, especially in women. On the fingers and palms, where warts tend to be deeper, liquid nitrogen often fails and I use surgical removal. Provided the freezing is superficial, scarring doesn't occur. The technique of liquid nitrogen therapy is discussed in Chapter 3.

Repeated liquid nitrogen treatment, sometimes combined with a home chemical-destruction approach, is one way of managing multiple warts.

When treating warts repeatedly with liquid nitrogen, you don't have to freeze deeply; repeated superficial freezings have been shown to be effective.

Cantharidin

Application of the blistering agent cantharidin (Cantharone) to warts has a discouragingly high failure rate. At times it makes the wart larger and doughnut-shaped. Since cantharidin is painless, I sometimes use it in treating multiple warts in children in spite of its drawbacks.

Apply a tiny amount of cantharidin in collodion precisely to the wart with a toothpick. Allow it to dry completely—about five minutes—and then cover it with a small piece of adhesive tape to improve penetration. The patient removes the tape when blistering occurs or after 48 hours, whichever is sooner. It's all right to get the treated area wet. No special precautions are necessary. If the degree of blistering is annoying, reassure the patient and be sure he leaves the area uncovered. Have the patient return in 10 to 14 days to assess the need for further treatment.

In treating small children, or warts located on cosmetically sensitive areas, it's a good idea to treat only one or a few warts and leave the warts uncovered. If the effect of uncovered cantharidin is inadequate, next time apply tape to the thoroughly dried cantharidin.

Chemical destruction

Chemical destruction is my preferred treatment for numerous warts. While surgical removal is excellent for one or a few common warts, it isn't practical when there are more than about five warts. Chemical destruction is painless; therefore I use it with small or anxious children even though they have only one or two warts that could be surgically removed in a fraction of the time needed to explain the chemical destruction treatment.

A self-treatment method using chemical destruction is the best answer for the patient with numerous ordinary warts, for it allows treatment of emerging warts as well as established ones. Please note that I did not claim chemical destruction is a "good" answer to the treatment of numerous warts; it's merely one of the best of our inadequate answers. Chemical self-treatment of warts is slow and requires perseverance and your encouragement.

Chemical wart destruction requires the repeated application of a moderately strong caustic such as salicylic acid, formalin, or lactic acid. One favorite is a salicylic acid-lactic acid mixture in flexible collodion marketed as Duofilm. Another useful formulation is a 40 per cent salicylic acid ointment. The addition of 10 per cent formalin increases the potency of the salicylic acid ointment. These caustics are used in a similar way and require:

1. Precise application to the wart with a toothpick or applicator. The caustic is applied most conveniently at bedtime. Duofilm comes with an applicator in the bottle. It should be allowed to dry until it forms a white film.
2. An occlusive covering for about eight hours for adequate penetration of the destructive agent. Occlusion is best accomplished by covering with wa-

terproof tape. The nonocclusive "paper" tapes are not suitable. The moisture-retaining and macerating effects of waterproof tape are desirable; there's no harm in the patient's getting the tape wet. If removal of the tape injures the surrounding skin, have the patient apply nail-polish remover between tape and skin when removing the tape. In patients with myriads of warts, occlusion with plastic film—plastic gloves on hands, Saran Wrap elsewhere—is a practical measure.

3. Mechanical removal of dead wart tissue using a pumice stone, tip of a metal nail file, curved scissors, or a similar instrument. This should be done after bathing, when the necrotic tissue will be soft. The mechanical removal step is crucial to effective treatment. Unfortunately, all too often it tends to be neglected. I frequently have to nag patients into performing necrotic tissue removal adequately.

4. Some flexibility in treatment. If destruction is inadequate, the patient should gradually increase the period of occlusion. If there's too much irritation, let the patient stop treatment for a day or two.

5. Patient compliance. Chemical wart destruction is self-treatment carried out at the physician's instruction. Patients must understand both the details of treatment and the need to continue it faithfully every day. While there's no substitute for your demonstrating the technique and explaining the need to continue treatment faithfully, a patient instruction sheet is also essential. I ask patients to read the instruction sheet on chemical destruction of warts once a day for three days to fix it in their minds.

6. Flexibility of follow-up. If a patient has numerous warts, have him return two to three weeks after starting treatment to check on progress. Patients often don't perform the treatment properly. Usually, as mentioned above, they're too timid about removing the dead wart tissue. For patients who are using chemical destruction on only one or two warts (usually they're small children), I use a more casual follow-up procedure, telling them to return only if no progress has been made in a month or if the wart is still present after three months of conscientious self-treatment.

The chemical destruction of warts can be combined with other modalities. In treating patients with multiple warts, I often combine light liquid nitrogen freezing with chemical destruction. The light freezing at the initial visit is not aimed to cure, but simply to start the destructive process and give the patient a psychological boost. I generally repeat light liquid nitrogen freezing at follow-up visits. In this situation, I don't know of a good substitute for liquid nitrogen. The stronger escharotics such as trichloroacetic acid, phenol, and the very destructive monochloroacetic acid are unpredictable and difficult to control. They often produce little effect and sometimes cause nasty scars. If liquid nitrogen is unavailable, pare down warts with a No. 15 Bard-Parker blade at follow-up visits.

Bleomycin

Injecting stubborn warts intralesionally with bleomycin (Blenoxane) is a new technique.[1] Bleomycin is a potent teratogen and expensive, and its solutions have limited stability. It's a treatment of last resort for stubborn plantar or periungual warts when there is *no* possibility of pregnancy.

Plantar warts

Plantar warts have a well-deserved reputation as a persistent, painful nuisance. Treatment often fails or is prolonged. The aim of therapy is to eradicate the wart without any scarring, for a plantar scar can be painful. Scars following electrodesiccation of plantar warts sometimes become painful only after a latent period of years.

Admittedly, many dermatologists claim scarring can be avoided if electrodesiccation is carefully performed. They're wrong. I've seen too many patients with painful electrodesiccation scars caused by dermatologists who have personally assured me that when *they* electrodesiccate plantar warts scarring never occurs. At times patients consult another physician, months or years after electrodesiccation of a plantar wart, complaining of a wart recurrence when the actual problem is a painful, hypertrophic scar (Figures C-46 and C-47). Never electrodesiccate a plantar wart.

Even careful surgical "scoop" removal may cause scarring. Sometimes, when a solitary plantar wart defies chemical destruction, careful surgical removal may be justified. If you undertake surgical removal, observe the same precautions recommended in surgically treating warts on cosmetically significant areas: Be gentle with your instruments and control bleeding with pressure and/or gelatin foam packing. Leave the electrodesiccator on the shelf, and do not use styptics such as Monsel's solution.

It's easy to state categorically what not to do in treating plantar warts. How to treat them is more difficult. Most perceptive clinicians use some type of chemical destruction.

There are innumerable formulas for chemical destruction of plantar warts. They all have about the same cure rate, so use the gentler approaches, which cause little or no pain. For one or a few plantar warts, I use Duofilm, 40 per cent salicylic acid ointment, or 10 per cent formalin in 40 per cent salicylic acid ointment. The patient applies the medicine at bedtime and covers it with tape overnight. Removal of dead wart tissue is essential.

Plantar warts are often painful. Suitable padding will relieve the pain by taking pressure off the wart. Commercially available corn pads are usually too small; I prefer a foam with one adhesive-coated surface (Dr. Scholl's Adhesive Foam). A piece of foam is cut large enough to cover either the entire heel or forepart of the foot, and a hole (or, if the wart is at the edge, a notch) corresponding to the position of the wart is cut into the foam. After sticking the pad on his foot, the patient stands for a few moments to promote adherence to his skin and then rolls a sock or stocking carefully over the pad.

The technique of making and applying the protective pad and the method to be used in treating the wart should be demonstrated to the patient in the office. A patient instruction sheet is also essential.

When there are numerous plantar warts, or in the presence of the extensive "mosaic" plantar wart, application of a chemical destructive to each wart is not practical. For multiple or very large plantar warts, dilute formalin soaks are useful. The patient is instructed to mix one tablespoon of commercial formalin (this contains 37 per cent formaldehyde) with one pint of cool water. The warty area of the sole is soaked in the diluted formalin for 10 to 15 minutes every night. The patient must systematically scrape off dead wart tissue after bathing. If there is soreness or itching, the treatment should be stopped, as irritation or sensitization occasionally occurs.

Flat warts

Flat warts are superficial, and gentle measures are indicated, especially as they often affect cosmetically sensitive areas (Figure C-48). For a few warts, very light liquid nitrogen freezing is useful. Cautious chemical destruction using Duofilm is often effective. Duofilm should first be used without occlusion. If the flat wart isn't in a cosmetically sensitive area, very gentle curettage can be tried.

With multiple flat warts, especially on the face, gentle peeling chemicals are widely used. For this purpose use one of the peeling acne preparations containing sulfur, salicylic acid, or resorcinol; an alternative is a retinoic acid acne topical (Retin-A). These preparations are designed to be used on the face and therefore will do no harm. The results with this technique are not spectacular; warts usually take a long time to disappear and sometimes resist the treatment completely. Counsel the patient and practice patience. Stress that the treatment is gradual and allow (if possible) two or three months between visits. Don't let the patient's frustration stampede you into using harsh measures that scar.

Acuminate warts

Acuminate warts, also known as moist or venereal warts, affect primarily the anogenital region. Although the term *venereal* is often used—and is appropriate, as many of these warts are related to sexual activity—I prefer to avoid *venereal* because of its connotation of serious disease. *Moist* describes both their location and their surface covering, which is softer and more permeable than the keratinous layer of warts elsewhere. This permeability explains the effectiveness of podophyllin (podophyllum resin) treatment.

Keep in mind that not all papular or verrucous lesions of the anogenital region are warts. The condyloma of secondary syphilis can mislead; a serologic test will settle the diagnosis. Malignancies—especially Bowen's disease—can closely resemble anogenital warts. Biopsy any atypical or persistent warty anogenital lesion.

Podophyllin doesn't work on all anogenital warts; it destroys only those warts on or close to mucous surfaces. Warts on the shaft of the penis, as well as scrotal warts, usually don't respond to podophyllin. Perianal warts, on the other hand, almost always do. Podophyllin can produce severe irritation. If there are many warts, treat a few as a trial. Use only a fraction of a drop (0.05

ml) at each treatment. If there's one huge wart, apply the podophyllin initially only to a portion.

CAUTION: Systemic symptoms from absorption of topical podophyllin are rare; fatalities from topical podophyllin have been reported, but have been *very* rare. In the published reports of toxicity, excessive quantities of podophyllin seem to have been employed. Because of possible teratogenicity, podophyllin should not be used in pregnant patients.

There are many techniques for using podophyllin. I paint acuminate warts with 20 per cent podophyllin tincture (alcoholic solution) on a cotton-tipped applicator. Most cotton-tipped applicators are too bulky; remove about 90 per cent of the cotton and tightly twirl the remainder around the stick. After dipping this slimmed-down applicator into the podophyllin tincture, allow it to dry in the air for a minute to thicken the mixture so it won't run onto normal tissue. Then apply a small amount of podophyllin precisely to the wart and allow at least three minutes for thorough drying.

Warn the patient to expect mild to moderate discomfort. Sitz baths in lukewarm water are advised if soreness develops. I also give the patient a sample tube of some nonmedicated lubricant (not a fluorinated corticosteroid) to apply to any sore warts. While some physicians advise patients to wash the medicine off six or eight hours after application, I have found this measure superfluous. There's also little use in applying petrolatum (Vaseline) to the surrounding normal skin prior to podophyllin applications.

If warts respond poorly to 20 per cent podophyllin tincture, I switch to a 20 per cent salicylic acid-20 per cent podophyllin tincture (must be compounded by a pharmacist). This causes stinging at the time of application and results in whitish discoloration of the treated wart. If warts resist this stronger medication (rare in perianal warts, but not uncommon in genital warts), alternative approaches are:

1. Snipping off the pedunculated acuminate wart under local lidocaine (Xylocaine) anesthesia with a serrated scissors as if it were a skin tag. This procedure is useful for one or just a few warts.
2. Liquid nitrogen freezing. Discard the applicator after use.
3. Application of cantharidin. The wart should be carefully dried before applying a tiny amount of cantharidin in collodion precisely to the wart with a toothpick. This can produce nasty blisters; if there are numerous warts, try it first on a few.

Periungual warts

Warts around the nails, or periungual warts, are especially frustrating to the wart therapist. Periungual warts of the posterior nail fold must be treated gently to avoid damage to the nail-forming matrix; otherwise a permanently deformed nail may result. When periungual warts grow under the nail to become subungual warts, the nail plate becomes a shield against treatment.

I don't know of any satisfactory treatment for periungual warts. The nondermatologist will do himself a favor by referring them to a specialist. When the patient has only one or two periungual warts, I prefer surgical "scoop" removal, provided the warts are not in the posterior nail fold. One frequently has to cut away a bit of nail to detect and remove subungual wart extension. About 40 per cent of periungual warts I treat this way recur, partly because it's difficult to find a precise cleavage plane between the wart and the pulpy fingertip tissue.

For multiple periungual warts, or those of the posterior nail fold, chemical destruction and/or repeated superficial liquid nitrogen freezing are my choices. These therapies don't produce scars and are often successful—although the many months that may be required will annoy both the patient and you. The patient must not only vigorously scrape away dead wart tissue but also steadily nibble away at the nail to expose subungual wart extensions to the destructive chemicals.

Reference

1. Cordero AA, Guglielmi HA, Woscoff A: The common wart: Intralesional treatment with bleomycin sulfate. *Cutis* 26:319, 1980

Appendix: Microscopic examination for fungus

Microscopic examination of skin scrapings for fungi is essential in dermatologic diagnosis. I do it daily. Fungal eruptions may closely resemble dermatitis. Most dermatologic diagnoses are made on clinical grounds; microscopy of skin scrapings provides objective information. A positive test clinches the diagnosis of fungal infection; a careful negative test makes it unlikely.

Many nondermatologists overdiagnose fungal infection. On the other hand, we all see cases of "stubborn dermatitis" in which the correct diagnosis of fungal infection is made only after the suspicious—or desperate—physician microscopically examines skin scrapings. Microscopy of potassium hydroxide-cleared skin scrapings—called a KOH exam—takes only a few minutes and is simple in principle. Doing it right takes expertise one can acquire only by practice. KOH exams should be performed by a physician or a well-trained assistant.

Technique

Using a sterile scalpel blade (No. 15 is convenient) moistened with tap water, scrape the edge of the lesion. Having the blade—or the skin—wet with water prevents scales from flying about. Transfer the scales to a slide that holds a small drop of water to prevent tissue loss. If there are blisters—not uncommon in tinea pedis—unroof them with the blade and a pointed forceps and put the blister roof on the slide.

After collecting the tissue, add one or two drops of 20 per cent KOH, put on a coverslip, and warm the slide gently for 15 to 30 seconds to hasten clearing. A wooden kitchen match is a simple source of heat. The addition of 40 per cent dimethylsulfoxide to the KOH solution accelerates clearing.

Examine the specimen using the low-power (10×) objective with the *condenser racked down* and the condenser diaphragm partly closed to provide minimum illumination. Lowering the condenser and closing the diaphragm are essential to accentuate the contrast between fungal elements (hyphae) and cellular borders. Use the 10× objective initially; the 3- to 5-power scanning objective is not adequate.

While searching the slide, raise and lower the focus. Changing the focus will help you spot hyphae—thin, often branching strands of uniform diameter that lighten when you raise the focus and darken when you lower it. When you've located a suspect element, switch to the high dry (43×) objective to confirm your finding. This will require raising the condenser and opening its diaphragm.

In candidiasis there are frequently thin pseudomycelia. It may be difficult to distinguish them from the hyphae seen in dermatophyte infection. You can tell whether you're looking at *Candida*, however, by the presence of groups of small, round yeast cells that glisten as you adjust the focus. On examination under the high dry objective these bodies are uniform in size (unlike oil droplets); some are budding.

Errors

Intercellular lines are the chief cause of error in microscopy of skin scrapings. They show as thin *single* lines whereas hyphae are strands with two borders. Hyphae have a smooth continuity, and intercellular lines a sort of zigzag appearance. The distinction is readily made by focusing up and down with the fine focus while using the high dry (43×) objective. Clothing fibers are another artifact. Fibers are irregular in width and often look frayed; hyphae are smooth and spaghetti-like.

Danger

KOH is caustic to tissues and microscopes. Keep it in a bottle distinctively different from any treatment-room medication bottles. It should be marked "Danger, Poison" and stored out of children's reach. If excess KOH spills over the edge of the slide, carefully wipe it off before placing the slide on the microscope stage.

Special situations

In tinea capitis, skin scrapings are usually negative; one must examine the hair to find fungi. Look for broken-off hairs; often the broken, infected hairs have a grayish coating. With pointed tweezers, pluck a broken-off hair and examine it microscopically after thorough clearing with KOH. An infected hair will have masses of small refractile bodies—the spores—in or around the hair shaft. The high dry (43×) objective is needed to delineate the spores. Spores are distinguished from oil droplets and other debris by their uniform small size.

In inflammatory ringworm, especially ringworm acquired from animals (zoophilic fungi), skin scrapings are frequently negative. Again, search for broken-off hairs, pluck them, and examine them under the microscope. Inflammation is one mechanism by which skin rids itself of fungi. It's more difficult to demonstrate fungi in an inflamed lesion than in one showing only some scaling and slight erythema, particularly in inflammatory ringworm.

Significance of positive and negative tests

A reliably performed positive KOH exam establishes the diagnosis of fungal infection. Unfortunately, a negative test doesn't exclude the possibility of fungus disease. While one can usually demonstrate fungi in noninflamed tinea pedis or tinea cruris, repeated scrapings may be necessary. Furthermore, in the presence of inflammation, even repeated KOH examinations are often negative. A negative KOH exam from an inflamed lesion means little. Repeat the microscopic examination in a few weeks, when the inflammation has subsided.

Illustrations in color

Where possible, the photographs on the following pages have been grouped to provide visual "mini" case histories. Each capsule is intended to make several teaching points. For example, Figures C-19 and C-20 convey three messages: (1) Herpes simplex in the beard area can be superficially mistaken for pyoderma; (2) the typical herpes picture consists of grouped blisters on an erythematous base; and (3) the disease can be transmitted by close contact. Following is a guide to these capsule histories:

C-1 to C-4: Wound closure with absorbable sutures
C-5 and C-6: Acne abscess
C-7: Excoriated acne
C-8 and C-9: Stretching the skin to detect basal-cell carcinoma
C-10 to C-12: Extensive basal-cell carcinoma
C-13: Basal-cell carcinoma mimicking dermatitis
C-14 and C-15: Technique of cyst removal
C-16: Nummular eczema and seborrheic keratoses
C-17 and C-18: Typical excoriated atopic dermatitis
C-19 and C-20: Herpes simplex
C-21: Impetigo
C-22: Molluscum contagiosum
C-23 and C-24: Shave removal of a nevus
C-25: Superficial spreading melanoma
C-26: Malignant melanoma arising from a lentigo maligna
C-27: Malignant melanoma arising from a congenital nevus
C-28 and C-29: Nickel allergy
C-30: *Rhus* dermatitis
C-31 and C-32: Palmar psoriasis
C-33 to C-35: The value of examining the entire patient in diagnosing psoriasis
C-36: Psoriasis of the ear
C-37: Psoriasis of the groin, mimicking tinea cruris
C-38: Rosacea leading to rhinophyma
C-39 to C-41: Treatment of papular rosaceaform dermatitis
C-42 and C-43: Scabies of the trunk and hand
C-44 and C-45: Burrows of the scabies mite
C-46 and C-47: Complication of electrodesiccation of a plantar wart
C-48: Flat warts mimicking acne

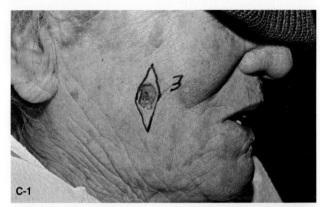

C-1

Figure C-1. Outline of excision of a squamous-cell carcinoma from the cheek of a 95-year-old woman.
Figure C-2. Closure of the incision with seven interrupted sutures of 5-0 plain gut.
Figure C-3. Wound covered with flesh-colored "paper" tape affixed with spirit gum adhesive. A gauze bandage was originally applied over the tape and removed 24 hours later. The tape must stay on for another 10 days.
Figure C-4. Result five weeks after surgery.

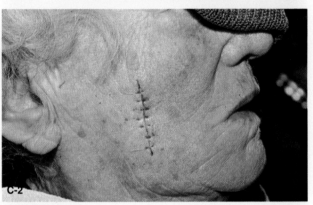

C-2

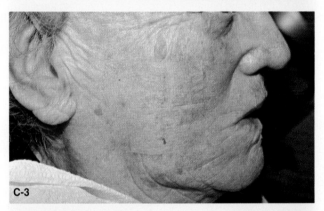

C-3

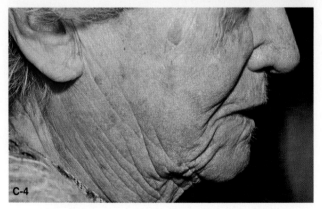

C-4

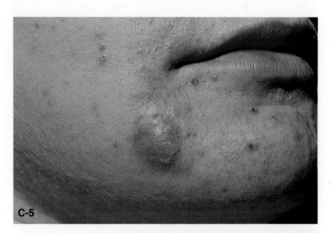

C-5

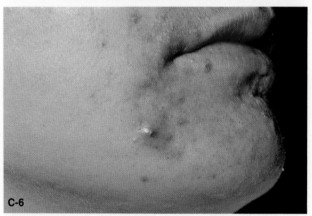

C-6

Figure C-5. Acne abscess on the chin of a woman.
Figure C-6. One week after intralesional injection of triamcinolone acetonide suspension, 2 mg/ml. The advantage of an intralesional corticosteroid is resolution without surgically induced scarring.

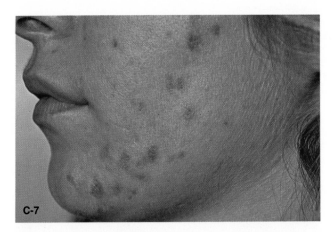

Figure C-7. Severely excoriated acne in a young woman. The lesions are mainly the result of her picking. Behavior modification is just as important as medication in suppressing this patient's acne.

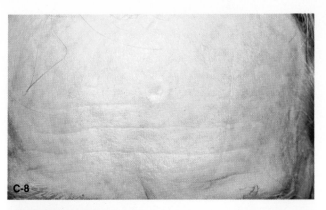

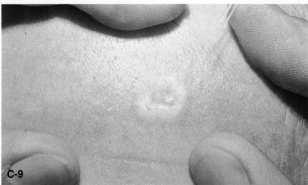

Figure C-8. Ill-defined depression on the forehead of a fair-skinned man.
Figure C-9. Closeup of the same lesion after the skin has been stretched to help delineate the margins, revealing this to be an infiltrating basal-cell carcinoma. Stretching the skin is a useful technique in examining skin tumors.

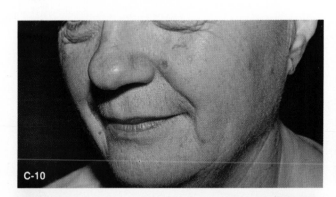

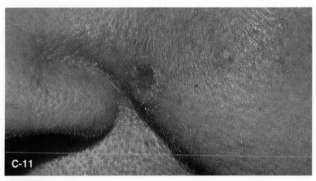

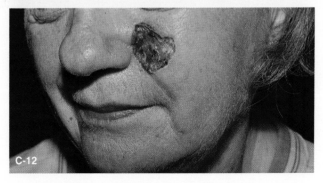

Figure C-10. Sharply demarcated papule clinically suggestive of basal-cell carcinoma. Biopsy confirmed the diagnosis.
Figure C-11. Closeup of the same basal-cell carcinoma before conventional surgical excision. Histology revealed basal-cell carcinoma infiltrating laterally on all margins, and the patient was referred for microscopically controlled excision.
Figure C-12. Extent of the defect after all strands of infiltrating basal-cell carcinoma had been traced out and removed by microscopically controlled excision. The lesion extended widely into clinically normal skin. Fortunately, this is uncommon, but it illustrates how tricky and dangerous basal-cell carcinoma can occasionally be.

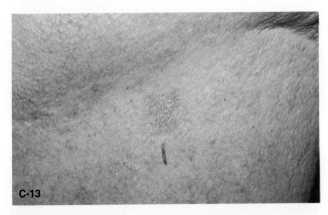

Figure C-13. Closeup of superficial basal-cell carcinoma of the upper neck (just above black line). Sometimes a stringlike, slightly pearly border suggests the correct diagnosis, but in this case the sign is absent and the lesion mimics dermatitis.

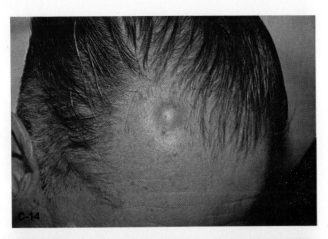

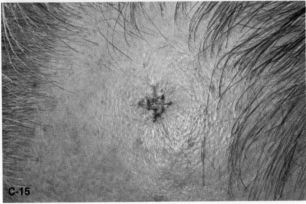

Figure C-14. A 14-mm cyst on the forehead of a man.
Figure C-15. Closeup after surgery. The cyst was incised through an 8-mm-long incision and deliberately ruptured, and the sac was dissected out as described in the text. The incision was closed with one vertical mattress suture and two interrupted sutures of 6-0 plain gut.

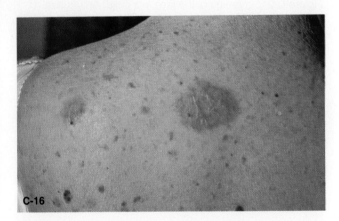

Figure C-16. Nonspecific nummular dermatitis of the back in a 72-year-old woman living alone. This is a common event in the elderly. The patient could not reach the lesions, so they were injected with a repository corticosteroid. Note the numerous seborrheic keratoses. Since they weren't bothering her, none were treated.

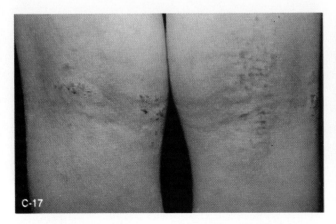

Figure C-17. Excoriated atopic dermatitis of the popliteal spaces—a typical location—in an 8-year-old child.

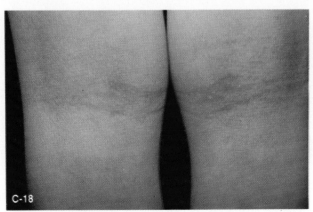

Figure C-18. Clearing of atopic dermatitis following 10 days of twice-daily application of a midstrength corticosteroid ointment. Avoidance of soap and lubrication with bath oil were also part of the treatment.

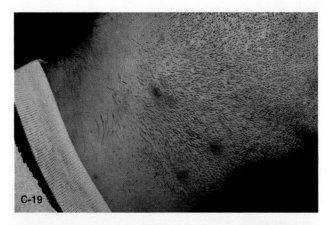

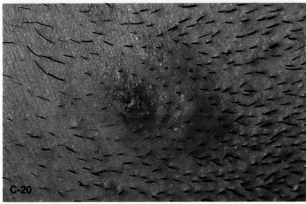

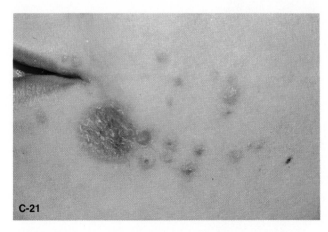

Figure C-21. Impetigo of the face in a child. An unusual number of intact blisters are evident. These are superficial and will soon rupture, leaving crusted patches, often with telltale scaling borders.

Figure C-19. Lesion that at first glance appears to be a bacterial infection (pyoderma) of the beard area—a common problem.
Figure C-20. Closeup of the same lesion, showing the typical picture of herpes simplex with grouped blisters on an erythematous, edematous base. The patient's girl friend had facial herpes simplex.

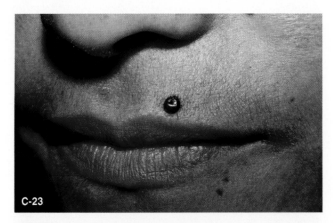

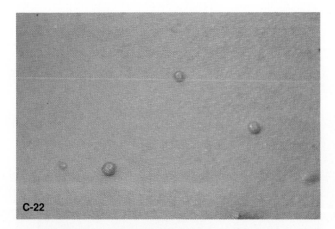

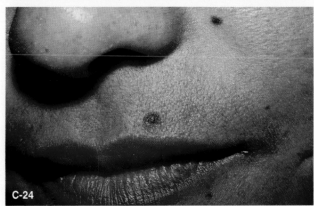

Figure C-22. Multiple lesions of molluscum contagiosum on the trunk. The lesions have a firm, waxy appearance, and the diagnostic central dell, or umbilication, is evident.

Figure C-23. Prominent, dark, benign-appearing nevus that worried the patient, a 21-year-old woman.
Figure C-24. Nevus after shave removal. The lesion is now flat and less noticeable, and shave removal provided a specimen for histology. Microscopy confirmed the impression of a benign compound nevus.

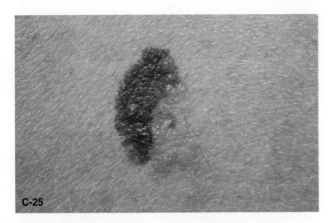

Figure C-25. Superficial spreading melanoma—the pigmented area at left—arising from a long-standing fleshy nevus of the back. The variation in color, irregular outline with notching in the lower portion, and recent color change made this lesion suspect and led to excisional biopsy.

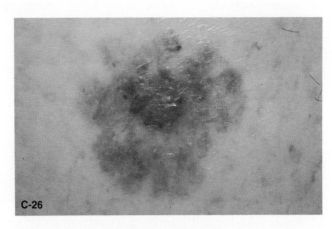

Figure C-26. Nodular malignant melanoma arising from a lentigo maligna. Note the irregular, notched border of the brownish lentigo maligna.

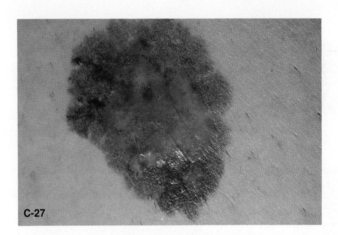

Figure C-27. Closeup of nodular malignant melanoma arising from a congenital nevus. The variegated coloration—bluish and reddish areas in a brown or black lesion—is a warning sign.

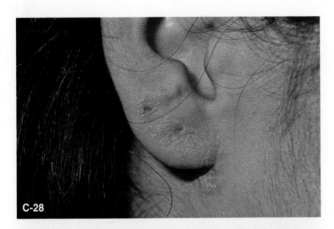

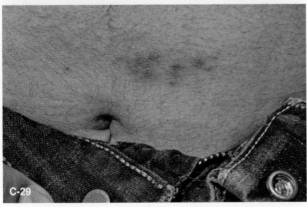

Figure C-28. Ear lobe dermatitis due to nickel allergy in a 23-year-old woman. Seborrheic dermatitis is another possible diagnosis.
Figure C-29. Dermatitis on the patient's abdomen corresponding to contact with the metal snaps of her blue jeans—a finding that strengthens the case for nickel dermatitis in this young woman. A positive patch test later proved the diagnosis.

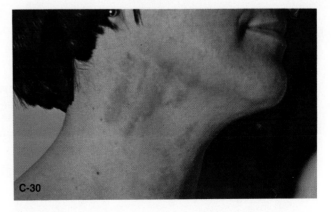

Figure C-30. Acute poison oak contact dermatitis on the neck of a young woman recently exposed to brush. Note the streaks of edematous dermatitis just beginning to vesiculate.

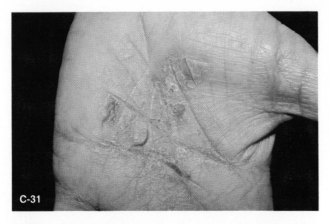

C-31

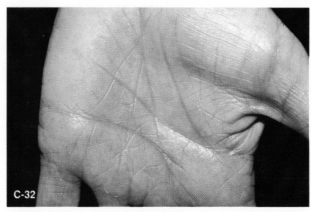

C-32

Figure C-31. Psoriasis presenting as hand dermatitis in a 52-year-old woman. Note the sharp demarcation of the lesions and the painful fissuring.
Figure C-32. Palmar psoriasis in the same patient after two weeks of treatment with a potent fluorinated corticosteroid at bedtime combined with daytime use of a medicated lubricant containing hydrocortisone. The skin's shiny, glazed appearance indicates early skin thinning and the need to phase out the fluorinated product.

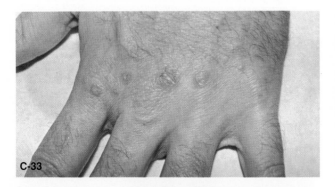

C-33

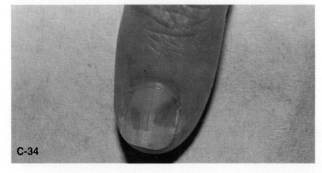

C-34

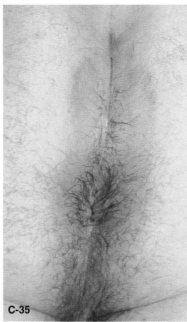

C-35

Figure C-33. Psoriasis of the dorsum of the hand. Mild rashes like these are easy to overlook. If you suspect psoriasis, examine the rest of the patient's skin.
Figure C-34. Psoriatic fingernail changes in the same patient: early distal oncholysis and, more proximally, a brownish "oil stain" color change heralding further oncholysis. These changes are often incorrectly attributed to a fungal infection.
Figure C-35. Typical perianal psoriasis in the same patient, extending up the gluteal cleft with fissuring. There's a superimposed irritation from an over-the-counter hemorrhoid ointment. This finding establishes the diagnosis of psoriasis and illustrates the value of examining the patient's entire skin.

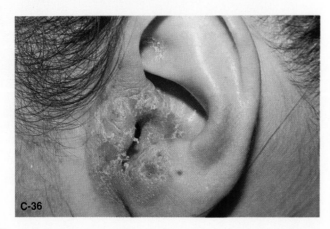

C-36

Figure C-36. Psoriasis of the ears, treated incorrectly for years as "chronic otitis externa."

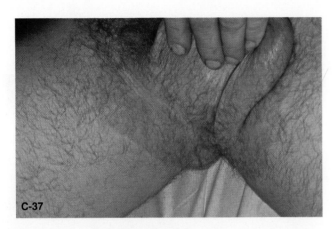

Figure C-37. Psoriasis of the groin, perfectly mimicking tinea cruris. Repeated skin scrapings were negative for fungi, and the eruption cleared with a mild topical corticosteroid.

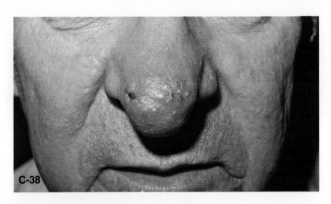

Figure C-38. Rosacea affecting primarily the nose, with swelling, pustules, and erythema. It has already led to rhinophyma. Tetracycline was prescribed and proved dramatically effective.

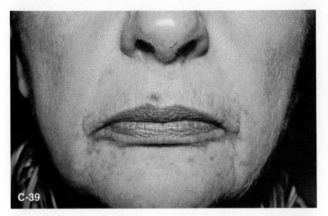

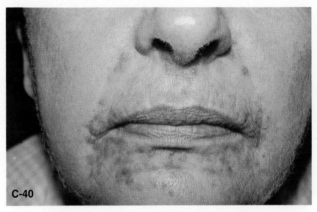

Figure C-39. Papular rosaceaform dermatitis. The patient, a 52-year-old woman, complained that her skin would temporarily improve, but never clear, with the many potent topical corticosteroids she had been given.
Figure C-40. Flare-up of rosacea in the same patient, as expected, one week after stopping treatment with corticosteroids and starting tetracycline. Tetracycline suppresses this disorder, but slowly.
Figure C-41. The same patient, after nine weeks of treatment with tetracycline. Her skin is perfectly clear.

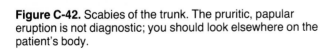

Figure C-42. Scabies of the trunk. The pruritic, papular eruption is not diagnostic; you should look elsewhere on the patient's body.

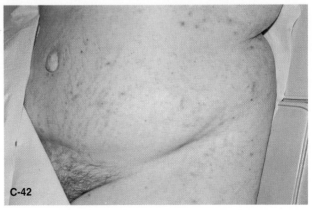

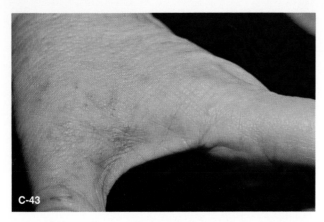

Figure C-43. Hand of the same patient as in Figure C-42. Papules, crusts, and small vesicles on the hands, especially the finger webs, should make you suspect scabies.

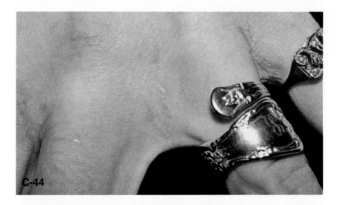

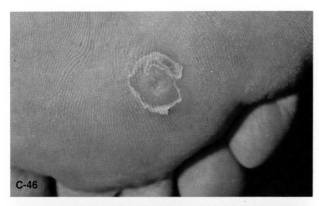

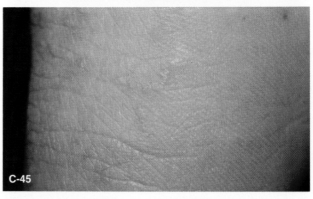

Figure C-44. Burrow of the adult female scabies mite in a finger web—the diagnostic finding. This one is unusually long and prominent.

Figure C-45. Multiple burrows on the same patient's wrist. The wavy shape and slightly scaly aspect help distinguish burrows from scratches. Despite these features, the burrows blend easily into the skin folds. Good lighting and low-power magnification are essential in the search for these burrows.

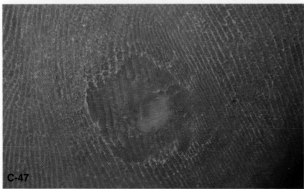

Figure C-46. Lesion on the plantar area treated for over 20 years as a supposed plantar wart after it had been "destroyed with an electric needle."

Figure C-47. Closeup after overlying hyperkeratosis was pared away, revealing a corn over a scar—the permanent sequela of destructive electrodesiccation over 20 years earlier. This is why I approach plantar warts gently, avoid surgery, and never electrodesiccate.

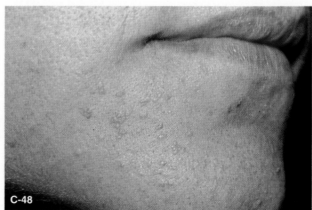

Figure C-48. Flat warts on the chin of an 18-year-old woman. These sometimes aren't recognized; this patient was told she had acne. Gentle peeling agents will avoid scarring and usually heal flat warts over a period of time.

Index

Patient Instruction Sheets

Contents

Acne

Acne is the term for the pimples and complexion problems that trouble many young people. Pimples occur mainly on the face, but often involve the neck, chest, back, and upper arms. Acne is only a skin problem and has nothing to do with your general health.

What causes acne?

Acne is caused by the oil glands of the skin breaking open. At puberty, the oil glands in the skin start producing an oily material called sebum. Sebum is discharged onto the skin's surface. Sometimes the wall of the oil gland breaks and spills the sebum within the skin. The sebum irritates the skin tissues and causes redness, swelling, and pus—in other words, a pimple.

Oil glands may become plugged and form blackheads and whiteheads. Blackheads are not caused by dirt. Removing blackheads will *not* prevent pimples. Blackheads and whiteheads are small nuisances. Try to ignore them.

In mild acne, only a few oil glands break open; in severe acne, many do. How easily oil glands do this seems to be "built into" you. Acne runs in families. It's impossible to prevent acne, since there's no way of changing your oil glands.

Age and acne

Acne usually begins mildly in the teens, gradually worsens, and then after a time improves. How long you will have acne is impossible to predict. Acne gets worse and improves by itself. There's usually no explanation for these ups and downs. Don't assume that because your acne gets worse, you've done something wrong. And, if your acne gets better briefly, it may not have happened because of treatment. In women, acne may worsen about the time of the menstrual period.

Skin hygiene

Dirt does *not* cause acne, despite what you may have been told. The oil on the skin's surface does no harm. Special soaps, astringents, abradants, and acne cleansers are a waste of money. Wash your face with ordinary soap and water only as much as you need to keep it clean. Too much washing and scrubbing can cause skin irritation. Cleanliness may be next to godliness, but it doesn't help acne.

Do not pick, squeeze, or otherwise manipulate your pimples, as it can leave scars.

Diet and acne

Foods do *not* cause acne. Many persons try all sorts of diets and are frustrated because they don't help. In some people, certain foods do make acne worse. The most common ones are chocolate, nuts, cola drinks, and root beer. A few people who drink large quantities of milk—over a quart daily—find that this worsens their acne. Aggravation of acne by food varies from person to person. Many acne patients can eat chocolate without trouble, while others find that even a few pieces of chocolate cause new pimples. Find out for yourself if the foods just mentioned aggravate your acne. Eliminate one for a few weeks and then test its effect by eating a large amount. If your skin improves when you stop eating a food and gets worse when you start eating it again, repeat the test. Acne has ups and downs of its own; make sure that the worsening isn't just a coincidence. If certain foods definitely worsen your acne, avoid them.

Nerves and acne

Acne is *not* caused by nerves and worry, but may become worse under stress such as examinations or pressure at work. These are usually mild, temporary flare-ups. Some persons react to stress by picking, squeezing, or rubbing their pimples, and this can make their acne worse.

Treatment

Unfortunately, there is no medical cure for acne, *although it can be controlled until you outgrow it.* This often takes years; therefore treatment may require many months or years.

The best current treatment for acne is antibiotics. They may be put on the skin or taken by mouth. Mild acne is often controlled by antibiotics applied to the skin. Antibiotics taken by mouth are usually needed in order to control moderate or severe acne.

Antibiotics do not remove blackheads and whiteheads. Certain other medicines put on the skin will help get rid of them for a while. These preparations may irritate the skin, and many patients find they're more trouble than they're worth. If you feel your blackheads and whiteheads are a real problem, discuss it with me. Otherwise you can safely ignore them. They can be hidden with a little water-based makeup.

Antibiotics applied to the skin

Antibiotics applied to acne skin are usually clear liquids. Many come in convenient "dab-on" applicator bottles. The liquid evaporates and leaves a thin film of invisible antibiotic on the skin. It is important to leave this film on your skin for several hours. Apply your antibiotic medicine in the morning *after* washing or shaving, and again at bedtime after washing. If you use makeup, put the antibiotic on first and let it dry before you put on the makeup. Apply the antibiotic medicine to the entire area of skin with acne, not just to a few pimples. Antibiotic lotions agree with most persons' skin, but some find them too drying. If that happens, we will prescribe an antibiotic cream.

Antibiotics taken by mouth

Tetracycline, erythromycin, and minocycline are among the internal antibiotics used in treating acne. Sometimes it's necessary to try several different antibiotics, or a combination, before acne is controlled.

Tetracycline is the most widely used antibiotic for acne. It helps about two out of three acne patients. Just how it works—and why it sometimes doesn't work—is not known. Tetracycline works slowly; you have to take it for about six weeks to find out whether it will help you. If you're better

after six weeks, the treatment will be continued since tetracycline controls your acne only while it's being taken. If your acne doesn't improve, the treatment will be changed.

Tetracycline should be taken with a full glass of water on an empty stomach since food, especially milk and dairy products, interferes with its action. It's simplest to take two capsules on arising and another two in the evening.

Tetracycline is remarkably safe and does not interfere with other medicines, except for iron and antacids. Tetracycline causes some persons to sunburn easily. If you notice that you're sunburning faster than usual, protect your skin with a sunscreen or clothing. Sun sensitivity is a problem mainly in the spring or summer, and when skiing. Women occasionally develop an annoying itch and discharge in the vagina. This can happen with any antibiotic. If it occurs, continue your medicine and telephone my office for treatment of the itch.

Sunshine

Sunlight benefits many acne patients, but also ages the skin. If sunlight improves your complexion, get moderate amounts of it. Don't sunburn or "bake" for hours. If the sun actually makes your acne worse, try to avoid heavy exposure. Don't bother with sunlamps. They can't duplicate natural sunlight and are worthless in treating acne.

Camouflage

Women may safely cover their acne with makeup or a foundation lotion. Use a water-based product. Wash the makeup off thoroughly at bedtime with soap and water. If you prefer, you may use a flesh-tinted acne lotion instead of makeup. Some men like to use an acne lotion to disguise prominent pimples.

Don't let your pimples get you down. They're a temporary cosmetic nuisance; try to live with them for a while. They won't interfere with your life unless you waste time worrying about them.

Actinic keratoses

What causes actinic keratoses?

Repeated, prolonged sun exposure causes skin damage, especially in fair-skinned persons. Sun-damaged skin becomes dry and wrinkled and may form rough, scaly spots called actinic keratoses. These rough spots remain on the skin even though the crust or scale is picked off. Treatment of an actinic keratosis requires removal of the defective skin cells. New skin then forms from the deeper skin cells, which have escaped sun damage.

Why treat actinic keratoses?

Actinic keratoses are *not* skin cancers. Because they may sometimes turn cancerous, however, they should be removed.

Treatment

Actinic keratoses can be removed surgically with scissors or a scraping instrument called a curette. Another way of destroying actinic keratoses is to freeze them with liquid nitrogen. Freezing causes blistering and shedding of the sun-damaged skin. Sometimes we're not sure whether the growth is harmless. When this occurs I prefer to cut the growth off and send it for microscopic analysis (biopsy). Healing after removal usually takes two to four weeks, depending on the size and location of the keratosis. Hands and legs heal more slowly than the face. The skin's final appearance is usually excellent.

When there are many keratoses, a useful treatment is the application of 5-fluorouracil (5-FU). The medication is rubbed on the keratoses for 10 to 20 days. 5-FU destroys sun-damaged skin cells. After three to five days the treated area starts to get raw. The applications are continued until your physician determines that you have the needed results. Healing starts when the 5-FU is stopped. 5-FU is effective in removing actinic keratoses from the face, but it often fails when used on the hands, forearms, or back.

Prevention

Sun damage is permanent. Once sun damage has progressed to the point where actinic keratoses develop, new keratoses may appear even without further sun exposure. You should avoid *excessive* sun exposure—but don't go overboard and deprive yourself of the pleasure of being outdoors. *Reasonable* sun protection should be your aim. It's described in a separate information sheet.

Alopecia areata

What causes alopecia areata?

In alopecia areata round patches of hair loss appear suddenly. The hair loss is often discovered by a barber or hairdresser. The hair-growing tissue stops making hair, and the hair then falls out from the roots. Why this happens is a mystery. Alopecia areata is not contagious, not caused by foods, not the result of nervousness. It sometimes runs in families.

Alopecia areata has three stages. First, there is sudden hair loss. Then the patches of hair loss may enlarge. Last, new hair grows back. This takes months—sometimes more than a year.

Treatment

Hair usually grows back by itself, but slowly. Sometimes the new hair is temporarily gray or white, but after a while the original color usually returns. The natural regrowth of hair can often be speeded up by injecting a cortisone medicine into the area of hair loss. The cortisone is injected into the skin. It acts only in the area where it has been injected. Unfortunately, there is no way of preventing new areas of hair loss. However, if new areas of hair loss appear, regrowth may be helped by injecting the cortisone.

Skin cancer
(basal-cell carcinoma)

What causes skin cancer?

The skin cancer (basal-cell carcinoma) for which you are being treated is common and *always curable.* Basal-cell cancers are the result of sun damage to the skin. Sunlight ages the skin cells, causing their growth to be disturbed. A basal-cell cancer begins as a small spot that grows slowly and relentlessly until treated. Basal-cell cancers enlarge steadily, but they *never* spread to distant parts of the body and *never* invade internal tissues.

Microscopic examination is necessary to determine whether a growth is cancerous. The tissue is examined by a pathologist in a medical laboratory.

Skin cancers are most common on the face. They're practically never found in areas such as the buttocks, which are protected from the sun by clothing. Skin cancers occur more often in people living in sunny areas like Texas, Arizona, and California than in areas receiving less sunshine, such as New England. Fair-skinned individuals are more prone to skin cancer than darker persons, since skin pigment protects the skin. Persons of African ancestry with very dark skins practically never get skin cancer.

Treatment

Basal-cell cancers are best treated early, when they're small, since it's simpler to remove a small growth than a large one. Surgical removal of basal-cell cancers is almost 100 per cent curative.

Very rarely, a cancer will grow back. In order to detect this rare event, the treated area should be checked periodically for five years. If you become concerned about the treated area or if other skin growths appear, please return to this office promptly.

Prevention

The skin-damaging effects of sunlight are permanent and build up slowly over time. Ordinary sun exposure and sunbathing produce gradual skin damage *even if sunburn is avoided.* As many as 10, 20, or more years can pass between the time of sun exposure and the time the skin shows signs of sun damage. Thus, teen-age sun worshippers often pay for their deep tans when they reach their 40s or 50s. There's no way of undoing sun damage. You can prevent further skin injury by using the sun-protective measures outlined in a separate information sheet. Be *reasonable* about sun protection. Don't go overboard and try to avoid the sun completely. The damage has already been done; a little more sun won't make things worse.

With the passage of time, skin-cancer patients are likely to develop additional skin cancers. If you notice a new growth, or a sore that doesn't heal or keeps coming back, be sure to have it examined.

This summary is intended to answer common questions about skin cancer. If you have additional questions, be sure to discuss them at your next visit.

Boils (furuncles)

What causes boils?

Boils are painful swellings of the skin caused by deep infection with staphylococcus bacteria. The bacteria enter the skin from the outside, usually through a hair opening. Boils begin as red, tender swellings. Later on the infection produces pus, which may ooze out through the skin. The source of the staph bacteria is usually not known. Most boils appear "out of the blue." Sometimes boils develop after exposure to someone with boils or another skin infection.

A few people have recurring boils. When this occurs, it's customary to test the urine and blood to check for any underlying disease, such as diabetes.

Treatment

Penicillin or other antibiotics taken by mouth usually speed healing in the early stages of a boil. If pus has formed, minor surgery to open the boil and drain the pus may be needed. Gentle heat, provided by a heating pad, hot water bottle, or lamp held close to the skin for 20 minutes three or four times a day, speeds up healing. Movement worsens a skin infection. You can help a boil heal by "resting" it—moving it as little as possible.

Putting medicine directly on a boil won't help it heal, since the medicine doesn't penetrate into the infected area. If pus is oozing out, a thin coat of antibiotic ointment (_____) and a Band-Aid over the boil will help keep the germs from spreading.

If your boil doesn't improve after treatment, please return, as a different antibiotic or minor surgery may be needed.

Cortisone ointments

What is a cortisone ointment?
Cortisone skin preparations in the form of ointments and salves contain hydrocortisone or a similar chemical. Actually, hydrocortisone is a natural chemical made by the body, but chemists have learned to manufacture stronger synthetic cortisones. Many skin medications contain these powerful synthetic cortisones.

Safety
Although cortisone taken by mouth can cause side effects, cortisone skin preparations are remarkably safe. They're even available without prescription in a $\frac{1}{2}$ per cent strength. Internal side effects from cortisone applied externally are rare, but you should check regularly with your doctor if the following conditions apply:

1. You are using strong cortisones over most of your body for many months.
2. Strong cortisones plus plastic covering, which increases penetration, are applied to much of the body surface.
3. Strong cortisones are used on *large* areas of a child or infant.

Local side effects
Strong cortisone medications may damage the skin to which they are applied, especially at skin-fold areas, fingertips, and the face. Skin thinning, or atrophy, is the most troublesome side effect: The stronger the cortisone, the greater the risk of atrophy, and the risk is increased when plastic covering also is used. Atrophy makes skin-fold sites (groin, rectal area, armpits) tender and raw. Cortisone atrophy of fingertip skin causes painful cracks. Cortisone atrophy of the face results in a flushed appearance with small blood vessels becoming noticeable.

Not every skin disorder responds magically to cortisones. They can worsen some diseases, such as athlete's foot, ringworm, and acne. Strong cortisones applied to the face may cause a red, pimply rash.

How to use cortisone ointments
Use a *small* amount of cortisone preparation and massage it gently into your skin. Ointment or salve left on the surface is wasted. Keep the medication away from your eyes. If eyelids are to be treated, use a clean fingertip and apply only a tiny amount of the preparation carefully, avoiding your eyes.

Summary
Cortisone ointments and salves are some of our safest and most effective skin medicines. Internal side effects are rare, but the skin—especially on the face and at skin-fold areas—can be damaged by strong cortisone preparations. Use them only under your doctor's supervision.

Cysts

What causes a cyst?

A cyst is a harmless, sac-like growth in the deeper layers of the skin. The cyst sac is filled with a soft, whitish brown material that sometimes oozes out onto the skin's surface. We don't know why cysts appear, nor do we know why some persons get many of them.

Cysts are a nuisance, but they *never* become cancerous or malignant. Occasionally germs get into the cyst and cause an infection that resembles a boil. When this happens, antibiotics taken by mouth and minor surgery performed in the office may be needed to relieve the pressure and discomfort.

Treatment

Small cysts—those $\frac{1}{4}$ inch in diameter or less—ordinarily don't need treatment unless they mar your appearance. Larger cysts are usually removed because of their size and the danger of infection.

Cysts are treated by making a small surgical opening into the skin and removing the sac. This small operation is done in the office. A local anesthetic is used to numb the skin. Stitches are often used to close the skin opening and are removed three to seven days later. Surgery usually cures cysts, but sometimes a cyst comes back and requires a second treatment.

Dermatitis

What causes dermatitis?

Dermatitis is a harmless but annoying rash. It results from a combination of causes and is not contagious. Think of dermatitis as skin "misbehaving."

Treatment

Dermatitis is treated by applying a cortisone-type medicine. Your skin should start to improve within a week; sometimes treatment takes longer. As long as you follow directions, cortisone medicines are safe to use on the skin until your rash clears up.

Skin suffering from dermatitis is easily irritated. Treat it gently. Since soap is irritating, keep it away from areas of dermatitis. Home remedies, over-the-counter medicines, and your neighbor's treatment suggestion rarely help and often make matters worse. Don't use them!

Please follow these directions:

1. Apply small amounts of cortisone to your skin as often as directed on the label. Massage it in gently but thoroughly.
2. Do not apply anything to your rash except (1) water, (2) the medicine prescribed for your dermatitis, and (3) white petrolatum (plain Vaseline). If your skin is dry, you may apply white petrolatum as often as you need to. Petrolatum is best used *after* you've applied the medicine. It may be most convenient to apply petrolatum sparingly at bedtime, when its greasiness is least objectionable.
3. Keep soap away from dermatitis. If you shower, it's all right to use a little soap on *normal* skin. Be sure to rinse it off well. If the dermatitis is widespread, you should shower or bathe with plain water and not use any soap.
4. Keep your skin well lubricated, using the cortisone and white petrolatum. When there is widespread dermatitis, lubrication with a bath oil *prescribed by the doctor* is convenient. The bath oil is applied sparingly with the fingers to the *entire* freshly dried skin after the bath or shower. Put a few drops of bath oil on your hands, spread it thinly, and repeat until the body is covered. A teaspoonful is enough for the whole body of an average adult.
5. Wool and other rough clothing may aggravate dermatitis. Wear something smooth and soft next to your skin.
6. If your dermatitis doesn't improve with these measures, please call and make an appointment.
7. Keep your medicines and this sheet even after your dermatitis has cleared because dermatitis tends to come back. If it does, resume the original treatment.

CAUTION: *Cortisone medicines are to be used only on dermatitis.* They may actually worsen other rashes such as athlete's foot or impetigo. Strong cortisone ointments may cause rashes when used on the face and may result in thinning of your skin when applied to skin-fold areas. Use your cortisone only for treating dermatitis, and only for the areas prescribed.

Atopic dermatitis (atopic eczema)

Atopic dermatitis, also called atopic eczema or just eczema, is the name given to a stubborn, itchy rash that occurs in certain persons with sensitive or irritable skin. Eczema is common in infants and young children, and may disappear before adulthood. Eczema may clear for years, only to reappear later—often on the hands.

What causes atopic dermatitis?

The cause is not known. It's the result of a built-in defect of the skin that tends to run in families. Eczema is not contagious and is not related to your general health. Atopic dermatitis is also called "constitutional eczema"; this name emphasizes the built-in aspect. Persons with eczema have skin that is dry and easily irritated by soap, detergents, and rough woolen clothing. Very hot or very cold weather often aggravates eczema. While certain allergies may worsen eczema, they don't cause it. Skin tests do *not* help, since eczema is *not* due to an allergy.

Treatment

Since eczema patients have a constitutional skin defect, no permanent cure is possible. Fortunately, we have effective ways of controlling eczema; most persons are able to live comfortably with their skin handicap.

Cortisone compounds applied to the skin are the best medicine for controlling eczema. Most cortisone salves can be used safely for years. When large areas of the body are treated with strong cortisone salves, periodic medical checkups are necessary. Certain cortisones should not be applied to the face, armpits, groin, or rectal area. In severe eczema, it's sometimes necessary to take cortisone by mouth; however, this is done only for short periods and under the close supervision of a doctor.

Cortisone is applied to the skin in the form of lotions, creams, or greasy ointments. When the skin is very dry, ointments are often best. Whatever preparation you use, be sure to use only a little and massage it in well. If you wish to have more vigorous treatment, apply the medicine more often. Always remember to use just a little.

Other medicines are sometimes used. For stubborn eczema, salves containing coal tar can be helpful. Coal tar smells and stains the clothes. You can minimize these nuisances by using it at bedtime.

In controlling your eczema, remember:

1. Keep your skin well lubricated. If your skin is too dry, use a greasy cortisone salve or apply a little white petrolatum (Vaseline) after you rub in your cortisone cream or lotion. Using a bath oil in the tub or putting it on right after toweling dry will help keep your skin sufficiently moist.

2. Keep soap away from your eczema. Soap irritates and dries the skin. Persons with eczema should avoid it. When bathing or showering, use plain water; limit soap to your face, armpits, genital area, and feet. If you must wash your hands frequently with soap, rinse them carefully and afterward apply a little cortisone cream or ointment.

3. Avoid overheating. Most persons with eczema find that hot weather and heavy sweating worsen their eczema. In hot weather wear cool, loose clothing, and try to stay in air-conditioned buildings.

4. Avoid direct skin contact with wool or similar rough clothing.

5. Avoid anything that definitely aggravates your eczema. If certain creams, makeups, perfumes, and so on cause itching or irritation, don't use them.

6. It's usually possible to find a treatment routine that lets you control your eczema. Most treatments involve cortisone ointments or creams. When properly applied, these medications can be used safely for years.

7. If your eczema worsens and you can't control it, please return so we can give you a different treatment.

Hand protection for hand dermatitis

Hand dermatitis (hand eczema is another name for the same thing) is common. Hand rashes usually result from a combination of (1) sensitive skin and (2) irritation or allergy from materials touched. Everyone's hands routinely touch irritating soaps and detergents several times a day. Add the raw foods, solvents, paints, oils, greases, acids, glues, and so on that most of us touch at work or in the home, and you can see that the skin of your hands takes a beating.

Not everyone gets hand dermatitis. Many lucky persons have "tough" skin, but, unfortunately, some persons have skin that's easily damaged. The result is dermatitis. Persons with hand dermatitis often have dermatitis elsewhere, and frequently blood relatives have hand dermatitis. We can't toughen your skin, but we have effective treatment to heal your dermatitis.

Skin protection is an important part of treatment. This instruction sheet gives you detailed directions on how to protect your hands. Please read it carefully every day for a week to fix these instructions in your mind.

1. Protect your hands from direct contact with soaps, detergents, scouring powders, and similar irritating chemicals by wearing waterproof, heavy-duty vinyl gloves. Heavy-duty vinyl gloves (such as Cyralon brand) are better than rubber gloves, since you may become allergic to rubber. Heavy-duty vinyl gloves are usually available at paint and hardware stores. Buy four or five pairs so they can be conveniently located in kitchen, bathroom, and laundry areas. If a glove develops a hole, *discard it immediately!* Wearing a glove with a hole is worse than wearing no gloves at all.

2. The waterproof, heavy-duty vinyl gloves may be lined or unlined. You should have enough waterproof gloves so that the insides of the gloves can dry between wearings.

3. Wear waterproof gloves while peeling and squeezing lemons, oranges, or grapefruit, peeling potatoes, and handling tomatoes.

4. Wear leather or heavy-duty fabric gloves when doing dry work and gardening. Dirty your gloves—not your hands. If you keep house for your family, scatter a dozen pairs of cheap cotton gloves about your home and use them while doing dry housework. When they get dirty, put them in the washing machine. Wash your gloves—not your hands.

5. If you have an automatic dishwasher, use it as much as possible. If you don't, let a member of your family do the dishes. Do your laundry by machine, not by hand.

6. Avoid direct contact with turpentine, paint thinner, paints, and floor, furniture, metal, and shoe polishes. They contain irritating solvents. When using them, wear heavy-duty waterproof gloves.

7. When washing your hands, use lukewarm water and very little mild soap. Rinse the soap off carefully and dry gently. All soaps are irritating. No soap is "gentle to your skin" except in the minds of advertising writers—so don't waste your money on special soaps or "soap-free" cleansers.

8. Rings often worsen dermatitis by trapping irritating materials beneath them. Remove your rings when doing housework and before washing your hands.

9. When outdoors in cold or windy weather, wear unlined leather gloves to protect your hands from drying and chapping.

10. Use only the prescribed medicines and lubricants. Do not use other lotions, creams, or medications—they may irritate your skin.

11. Protect your hands for at least four months *after* your dermatitis has healed. It takes a long time for skin to recover, and unless you're careful the dermatitis may recur.

There is no fast, "magic" treatment for hand dermatitis. Your skin must be given a rest from irritation. Follow these instructions carefully.

Overnight plastic occlusion for hand dermatitis

Covering skin overnight with plastic increases the penetration and effectiveness of cortisone medicines. For hand dermatitis, you should wear plastic gloves overnight after applying a cortisone to your rash. You will receive a special cortisone to be used *only at bedtime.* Please follow these directions carefully.

1. At bedtime, apply _____
(a cortisone) thinly to the rash areas only. Do *not* apply it to normal skin. Then put on the plastic gloves; take them off in the morning. The plastic gloves recommended are B-P disposable vinyl examining gloves; they can be used again for a few nights or until they develop holes. They are made in four sizes; your proper size is: Small   Medium   Large   Extra large. If your drugstore doesn't stock them, our receptionist can tell you where to buy them.
2. At first, wearing the plastic gloves may be a bit uncomfortable. It may take a few days to get used to them.
3. The cortisone ointment-plastic glove treatment can make your skin become thin. You should use it exactly as directed on this sheet. It's important to apply the cortisone medicine *only to the rash* when using plastic gloves. Do *not* apply the cortisone medicine to normal skin. If your fingertips are normal, cut the fingertips off your gloves, as the plastic covering softens skin. If your rash is on only one or two fingers, cut the proper number of fingers from a plastic glove and hold them in place with a nonirritating paper tape.
4. During the day, follow the printed hand dermatitis treatment and hand protection instructions. Apply the daytime lubricant thinly and often to the entire skin of both hands.
5. Keep your follow-up appointment. You will need an appointment 7 to 10 days after starting the cortisone-plastic covering treatment.
6. CAUTION: *Strong cortisones covered with plastic may cause your skin to thin and crack easily.* To prevent this, be sure to use the cortisone-plastic glove treatment less often as soon as directed.
7. Follow these instructions exactly until your next appointment. The cortisone-plastic covering treatment should be used only under medical supervision.

Hand dermatitis treatment

1. The most important part of your treatment is to apply a cortisone medicine to your hands many times a day. You should apply the medicine after each hand washing and as often at other times as possible—at least 15 times each day. Apply the medicine very thinly to the rash and massage it in well. If you wish, you can apply the medicine to your whole hand like a hand cream. The medicine may be a lotion, cream, or ointment.

2. Do *not* apply any cream, lotion, or ointment to your hands except the one prescribed for you. One exception: If your skin is still too dry, you may apply plain white petrolatum (Vaseline) thinly *after* rubbing in your medicine.

3. When washing your hands, use lukewarm water and a very small amount of mild soap. Rinse the soap off well and dry gently. Then apply a little medicine and massage it in well.

4. Pamper your hands by following the hand protection instructions.

5. When your rash is *much* better, you may use the medicine less often. However, you should apply the medicine at least four times a day until your skin has healed completely.

6. Continue applying the medicine until your skin is completely normal. Pamper your hands for at least four months after healing. It takes a long time for skin to recover from prolonged inflammation.

7. Hand dermatitis is stubborn. If your hand rash improves at first and then worsens, it usually means you need to use your medicine more often.

8. Hand dermatitis often recurs. If your hand rash comes back, you need to apply the medicine often and pamper your hands.

9. Cortisones keep for years at room temperature. As long as the prescriptions are refillable, take the *original container* to your pharmacist for a refill when you need more medicine. If you've used up all the authorized refills, please make an appointment for a checkup.

10. If your rash doesn't clear up, please return to this office so we can re-evaluate your treatment.

Seborrheic dermatitis

Seborrheic dermatitis is a common, harmless, scaling rash that sometimes itches. Dandruff is seborrheic dermatitis of the scalp. Seborrheic dermatitis may also occur on the eyebrows, eyelid edges, ears, the skin near the nose, and such skin-fold areas as the armpits and groin. Sometimes seborrheic dermatitis produces round, scaling patches on the middle of the chest or scales on the back.

What causes seborrheic dermatitis?
Seborrheic dermatitis results from skin not growing properly. The cause is not known. Seborrheic dermatitis is *not* related to diet and is *not* contagious. Nervous stress and any physical illness tend to worsen seborrheic dermatitis, but don't cause it.

Seborrheic dermatitis may appear at any age, either gradually or suddenly. It tends to run in families. Seborrheic dermatitis may last for many years and may disappear by itself. Often it gets better or worse without any apparent reason.

Treatment
There is no cure for seborrheic dermatitis. However, we can keep this nuisance under control. The treatment of seborrheic dermatitis depends on what part of the body is involved. Dandruff—seborrheic dermatitis of the scalp—can usually be controlled by washing your hair often with medicated shampoos. Sometimes it's also necessary to use lotions or gels containing tar or cortisone. Remember that dandruff is a harmless nuisance. It does *not* cause hair loss.

In areas of smooth skin such as the face and ears, cortisone-containing creams, lotions, or ointments are effective. Cortisones applied to limited areas of skin do not affect your general health.

Once seborrheic dermatitis is under control, gradually use your medicines less and less. It may even be possible to stop the medicines completely, but occasional treatment is usually needed. Seborrheic dermatitis has a way of returning. If it does, resume the original treatment. If your seborrheic dermatitis isn't controlled by the treatment prescribed, please return for further evaluation.

Dermatofibromas

What causes a dermatofibroma?
A dermatofibroma is a round, brownish to purple growth commonly found on the legs and arms. Dermatofibromas contain scar tissue and feel like hard lumps in the skin. We don't know why people grow dermatofibromas. Some may be caused by insect bites. They are harmless and never turn cancerous.

Treatment
Dermatofibromas are best ignored. Sometimes, if the diagnosis is not certain, a piece may be removed for tissue analysis (biopsy). Dermatofibromas can be removed surgically, but since they are deep, this usually leaves an unsightly scar. When a dermatofibroma becomes bothersome—for instance, gets in the way of leg shaving or is irritated by clothing—it can be flattened by freezing with liquid nitrogen.

Liquid nitrogen freezing destroys only the upper part of the growth. Therefore, the dermatofibroma, after some years, may again become noticeable. Usually any regrowth is slight and can be handled by another freezing. If there is any unusual change or marked regrowth of a dermatofibroma, please return.

Dry skin (asteatosis, xerosis)

What causes dry skin?

Dry skin is a problem for many people, especially in cool weather when the air is dry. Dry air causes the skin to lose moisture and then chap and crack. These chapped, cracked areas may become irritated and itchy. The dry skin rash sometimes forms round patches that resemble ringworm.

Treatment

Skin lubrication

Treatment is intended to restore moisture to your skin. Water will briefly moisturize your skin, but the moisture is soon lost by evaporation. Lotions, creams, and ointments provide an oil coating that prevents water evaporation.

Bath oils are an effective way of preventing skin moisture loss. You can put bath oil on your freshly dried skin after a shower or bath or add it directly to the bath water (CAUTION: *Slippery tub!*). When applying bath oil directly to your skin, pour a small amount into your hands and then spread it onto your slightly damp skin immediately after toweling. To avoid feeling greasy, use just a little. A teaspoonful is enough for the entire body of an average adult. If you prefer to use a bath oil in the tub, add about a tablespoonful to the bath water and soak for 10 to 20 minutes. Do not use soap; you will get clean by soaking in the oil-water combination. Afterward, pat yourself dry with a towel; enough bath oil will remain on your skin to prevent moisture loss. There are many excellent bath oils on the market. Some of them are

---

If you prefer not to use a bath oil, you can use moisturizing creams, lubricating lotions, mineral oil, or plain petrolatum (Vaseline) with good results. Salad or cooking oil will give your clothes an unpleasant odor. Any lubricant is best applied after your skin has been wet, so as to trap and hold moisture. Mineral oil should not be added to the bath, as it doesn't mix with water as the commercial bath oils do.

Treating dry skin rash

When dry skin has developed into a rash that itches, a cortisone cream or ointment usually brings quick relief. The cortisone is applied thinly to the rash and massaged in well, usually at bedtime, after bathing, and one or two other times during the day. As the rash improves, the cortisone is used less often. Occasionally rashes are severe enough to require a few days of oral medication.

Soap
Soap is bad for dry skin. It removes skin oils needed to hold in moisture. Soap should *not* be used on dry skin. Most of us use far too much soap; actually, plain water is often enough for a shower or bath. If you can't live without soap, it's all right to use a *little* soap (rinsed off well) for your face, feet, armpits, and groin.

Bathing
Persons with dry skin may bathe or shower once daily—but not oftener. Remember two things: (1) Use no soap on dry skin areas; (2) lubricate your skin using one of the methods described on this sheet.

Long-term control
Dry skin is usually a long-term problem that recurs often, especially in winter. When you notice your skin getting dry, resume your lubricating routine and carefully avoid the use of soap. If the itchy dry-skin rash returns, use both the lubricating routine and the prescription cortisone cream or ointment.

5-Fluorouracil treatment

5-Fluorouracil (abbreviated 5-FU) has the ability to destroy sun-damaged skin cells. Applying 5-FU to the skin removes the rough spots resulting from sun damage (actinic keratoses). The skin is then smoother and more youthful-looking.

Apply 5-FU three times a day to the skin needing treatment. You may feel stinging or burning when you put 5-FU on your skin. This is normal. Three to five days after you start using 5-FU, your sun-damaged skin will become red and irritated. As you continue treatment, sores and crusts will appear. These raw areas result from the destruction of defective skin cells. They're a necessary part of 5-FU treatment.

You should be seen 10 to 12 days after starting treatment to check on your progress and determine how long to continue using 5-FU. When treatment is stopped, your skin will heal rapidly; in two or three weeks healthy new skin will have replaced the sun-damaged skin destroyed by the 5-FU. After healing, the treated areas will be redder than normal; this redness will gradually fade in the next few months.

Directions for use

1. Treat the following areas with 5-FU: _____

_____

2. Three times daily apply the medicine very thinly to the treatment area with your fingertip and massage it in well.

3. Afterward, rinse your finger thoroughly with water.

4. Do *not* get 5-FU into your eyes, and do *not* use it on your eyelids.

5. Keep 5-FU *off* your lips.

6. Use 5-FU with care in the area between the nose and cheeks, since the medicine may irritate the folds around your nostrils.

7. Do *not* sunbathe while using 5-FU.

8. If you wish, you may wash the area that is to be treated with plain water *before* applying 5-FU.

9. You may use makeup; be sure to apply the 5-FU before putting on makeup.

10. If you notice any unusual or severe reaction, stop the medicine and contact my office.

11. After you've been instructed to stop using the 5-FU, apply plain white petrolatum (Vaseline) thinly to raw and crusted areas at bedtime. This helps healing. Stop the petrolatum when the crusts and scabs have healed.

12. CAUTION: *5-Fluorouracil is a powerful, destructive medication and must be used exactly as directed.* Keep it away from your eyes and mouth. Keep your 5-FU locked up so other people can't mistakenly use it to treat a rash.

Fragile skin bleeding

What causes fragile skin bleeding?

Easy bruising and bleeding into the skin of the tops of the hands and forearms occurs in many middle-aged and older people, especially if their skin is fair. This easy bleeding—which can occur without apparent injury—is a result of the skin's being made thin and fragile by years of sunlight exposure. It is *not* the result of a blood disorder or internal disease. The fact that bleeding occurs only on the sun-damaged areas of the hands and forearms, and never on the covered parts of the body, clearly shows that it results from local skin damage.

Sun exposure over the years, even without sunburning, has thinned your skin and damaged its supporting fibers. These sun-damaged fibers can no longer adequately support your skin and its blood vessels. Even slight movement may cause an unsupported blood vessel to break. This releases blood into the skin and leaves unsightly purplish marks.

Treatment

Fragile skin bleeding is a harmless nuisance. The skin damage produced by sunlight is permanent, and for that reason we have no treatment for your problem. You can prevent further sun damage by using the sun-protective measures described in a separate instruction sheet.

Herpes simplex

What causes herpes simplex?

Herpes simplex, commonly called cold sores or fever blisters, may occur once or return again and again. It's caused by the herpes hominis virus. There are two kinds of herpes virus, type 1 and type 2. Type 1 virus causes the cold sores so common on the lips and face. Herpes of the genital area is usually caused by type 2 virus.

Herpes simplex begins as a group of small red bumps that blister. You may have noticed itching or discomfort before the rash appeared. The blisters begin to dry up after a few days and form yellow crusts. The crusts gradually fall off and leave slowly fading red areas. The whole process takes about 10 to 14 days. No scars form.

These mild symptoms are typical of *recurring* herpes simplex. The very first infection with type 1 herpes virus usually happens in childhood. It may go unrecognized, but often it causes fever, general illness, and much local soreness. Once you've had a herpes simplex infection, the virus becomes permanently established in your nerve tissue. Recurring herpes results from activation of this virus. Between attacks it lives quietly in nerve tissue.

Fever and sun exposure are the most common factors triggering type 1 herpes simplex virus. That's when cold sores or fever blisters break out. Often the virus becomes activated without any apparent reason.

Contagion

Like most other viruses, herpes simplex virus is contagious to people who have never had the infection before. Anyone who's had a fever blister or cold sore on the face is resistant to type 1 virus. Herpes simplex type 1 virus is not very contagious. Close contact such as kissing is necessary to transmit the infection.

Genital herpes (type 2) is usually spread through sexual intercourse and is essentially a disease of adults. It's also contagious when in the active stages. Recurring herpes is not a reinfection, but activation of virus present in a quiet form in nerve tissue.

Treatment

Unfortunately, we have no effective treatment for herpes simplex infections. Herpes simplex heals by itself in about 10 days. The amount of time depends on the size of the blisters and their location. Two simple remedies will make you more comfortable while you're getting over herpes:

1. While there is oozing and crusting, use dilute vinegar compresses. Mix two tablespoons of white vinegar with a quart of lukewarm water. Apply this diluted vinegar solution to your blisters with a clean cloth for 10 to 15 minutes two or three times a day.

2. Later on, when the blisters become yellow and crusted, you can relieve any cracking and dryness with small amounts of plain white petrolatum (Vaseline).

Recurring herpes is usually only an uncomfortable nuisance. One exception is herpes of the eye. Since it may lead to eye damage, you should see an eye doctor (ophthalmologist) immediately. Fortunately, eye involvement is rare with herpes simplex. Herpes simplex *around* the eye is *not* dangerous unless it involves the eye.

Prevention

Herpes simplex is unpredictable. It may attack every few weeks for months, then not come back for years. Vitamins, repeated smallpox vaccinations, herpes vaccines, dye and light treatments, and antiviral drugs applied to the skin have all been tried. Some of these remedies may have unpleasant side effects; all are worthless. Recurring herpes can be very distressing. Fortunately, attacks of genital herpes gradually become less frequent. We have to face the unfortunate fact that as yet there's simply no way to prevent recurring herpes simplex—with one exception.

Prevention of recurring herpes simplex is sometimes possible when attacks are triggered by sunlight. If sunlight acts as an activator for your herpes simplex, you should use a sunscreen on and around your lips when you go outdoors. You can use a heavily pigmented lipstick or a colorless sunscreening lip pomade

(_____)

available over the counter on your lips, and a sunscreen such as

_____

on the skin around your lips.

Summary

Fever blisters or cold sores are a harmless infection caused by the herpes hominis virus. There is no effective treatment for the rash. Fortunately, it heals by itself without leaving scars. Sometimes repeated attacks can be prevented if a triggering factor, such as sunlight, can be found and avoided. Herpes simplex is moderately contagious to people who have never had the infection.

Herpes zoster (shingles)

What causes shingles?

Shingles (herpes zoster) is a nerve infection caused by the chicken-pox virus. Shingles results from activation of chicken-pox virus that has remained in your body since you had chicken pox—perhaps many years ago. The virus activation is limited to a nerve root. That accounts for the pattern of the rash, which always stops at the body's midline. The nerve involvement explains the stinging, burning, or pain common in shingles. Some patients have discomfort before the rash appears.

The rash of shingles begins as red patches that soon develop blisters. The blisters may remain small or can become large. They heal in two to four weeks. They may leave some scars.

Many patients mistakenly believe that "nervousness" causes shingles. This is wrong; shingles is a viral infection of a nerve and has nothing at all to do with being "nervous."

Contagion

You don't have to quarantine yourself. Until your rash has healed, however, you should keep away from persons who have never had chicken pox. Small children or infants can catch chicken pox from someone with shingles. Persons whose resistance to infection is lowered by illness or certain medications, such as cortisone, can also catch shingles. Contact with healthy adults appears safe.

Treatment

There is no antibiotic or other drug effective against the chicken-pox virus. Therefore, in treating shingles, you can only be kept comfortable while nature does the healing. If you have feelings of burning or discomfort, take aspirin or a similar mild painkiller.

If you have much pain, you can be given a prescription painkiller to take until the pain subsides. The pain is caused by neuritis—inflammation of a nerve. Cortisone taken by mouth shortens this neuritis and is often prescribed for it. The blistering rash usually clears up in a few weeks. The discomfort may last longer.

Don't open your blisters. You should compress the blisters or crusts for 10 minutes twice daily with a mixture of one-quarter cup of white vinegar and two quarts of lukewarm water. Later, when the crusts and scabs are separating, your skin may become dry, tense, and cracked. If that happens, rub on a small amount of white petrolatum (plain Vaseline) three or four times a day.

Hives (urticaria)

Hives are itching red welts or small bumps that last from 15 minutes to several hours. They usually appear suddenly and leave no trace when they disappear. Crops of hives may appear several times a day. They may come and go for days or weeks, sometimes longer. Hives are harmless except when they cause throat swelling; this is rare but requires immediate treatment.

What causes hives?

Hives may be caused by something taken internally, most often a medicine such as penicillin or aspirin. Sometimes foods cause hives; shellfish and strawberries are well-known examples. Hives are sometimes caused by infections such as infectious mononucleosis or are the result of an internal disease. Occasionally physical agents such as pressure or cold can cause hives. Often the cause can't be found. Fortunately, we can usually treat hives successfully—even though their cause may remain a mystery.

Treatment

In treating your hives, we try to find their cause. Medicine is prescribed to control the rash and itching.

Since medicines are the commonest cause of hives, please list all the medicines you've been taking—including headache tablets, allergy pills, medicines for stomach discomfort, laxatives, tranquilizers, cough medicines, painkillers. Think for a minute of what your medicine cabinet contains. List any unusual foods you ate in the two days before the hives first appeared. Have you had any recent illnesses?

Answers to these questions may help find the cause of your hives. Meanwhile, you'll be given medicines to control them.

Hives are usually controlled with antihistamines. Often one type of antihistamine is prescribed for daytime use, and a different antihistamine for bedtime. CAUTION: *Antihistamines sometimes cause drowsiness; if you feel sleepy, don't drive.* Don't drink alcoholic beverages when taking antihistamines.

Injections of epinephrine (Adrenalin) may be used for treatment of severe hives. Sometimes epinephrine-like medicines taken by mouth are used in combination with antihistamines. If these drugs don't stop hives, it's likely that cortisone will.

Hives usually improve with medicines in 24 hours or less. If you are not better within 24 hours, call my office.

Medicines applied to your skin—lotions, creams, sprays, and so on—won't help your hives. However, cooling the skin often relieves severe itching. A cold shower is the simplest way; if your hives are confined to a small area, an ice pack is useful. Since warmth worsens itching, avoid overheating and hot baths.

When your hives have cleared up, keep taking the medicines in the same way for two more days. Once you've been free of hives for two days, *gradually* take less and less of your medicines over the next seven or eight days. If hives come back while you're tapering off the medicines, resume the original amount until the hives disappear. It's a good idea to take the medicines for about 10 days after the hives have cleared up while your body eliminates their cause.

While hives usually clear quickly with treatment, they can be stubborn and we may have to try different medicines. Sometimes the amount of medicine needs to be increased. If your hives don't go away in a few days, or if they last more than three weeks, call my office.

Impetigo

What causes impetigo?

Impetigo is a skin infection caused by germs. It's most common in children and is contagious. Impetigo forms round, crusted, oozing spots that grow larger day by day. The hands and face are the favorite locations for impetigo, but it often appears on other parts of the body.

How does one get impetigo? While the germs causing impetigo may have been caught from someone else with impetigo or boils, impetigo usually begins out of the blue without any apparent source of infection.

Treatment

Antibiotics taken by mouth usually clear up impetigo in four to five days. It's most important for the antibiotic to be taken faithfully until the prescribed supply is *completely used up*. In addition, an antibiotic ointment should be applied thinly four times daily. ointment is advised and can be purchased without a prescription.

Crusts should be removed before the ointment is applied. Soak a soft, clean cloth in a mixture of one-half cup of white vinegar and a quart of lukewarm water. Press this cloth on the crusts for 10 to 15 minutes three or four times a day for as long as you see crusting or oozing. Then gently wipe off the crusts and smear on a little antibiotic ointment. You can stop soaking the impetigo when crusts no longer form. When the skin has healed, stop the antibiotic ointment.

Contagion

Impetigo is contagious when there is crusting or oozing. While it's contagious, take the following precautions:

1. Patients should avoid close contact with other people.
2. Children should be kept home from school for one or two days.
3. Use separate towels for the patient. His towels, pillowcases, and sheets should be changed after the first day of treatment. The patient's clothing should be changed and laundered daily for the first two days.

All these measures are only needed during the contagious—crusting or oozing—stage of impetigo. Usually the contagious period ends within two days after treatment starts. Then children can return to school and special laundering and other precautions can be stopped. If the impetigo doesn't heal in one week, please return for evaluation.

Keloids

A keloid is a greatly enlarged scar that projects above the skin surface. Skin heals by formation of scar tissue, which at first is often red and somewhat prominent. With the passage of months a scar usually becomes flat. Unfortunately, sometimes scars enlarge to form firm, smooth, hard growths called keloids.

What is a keloid?
No one knows why keloids form. While most persons never form keloids, others develop them after minor injuries and even insect bites or pimples. Keloids may form on any part of the body, although the upper chest and upper back are especially prone to keloid formation. Dark-skinned persons form keloids more easily than Caucasians.

Keloids are a cosmetic nuisance and never become malignant.

Treatment
We have no satisfactory treatment for keloids. Surgical removal of a keloid usually results in a second keloid even worse than the first. The best treatment is to inject a long-acting cortisone into the keloid itself. After injection with cortisone, the keloid usually becomes less noticeable and flattens in two to three months. The injection can be repeated after two or three months if necessary.

Moles

What causes moles?

Moles are harmless skin growths that may be flat or protruding. They vary in color from pink flesh tones to dark brown or black. Everyone has moles; some of us have a lot, others have only a few. The number depends on our genes. Moles sometimes appear in "crops," especially during the early teens.

Moles begin to grow in infancy. New ones can develop at any age. Once a mole appears, it usually stays for life without becoming a medical problem. A growing or changing mole *in a youngster* is almost always harmless. On the other hand, if an adult's mole markedly changes in color or size, or bleeds, it should be checked by a physician.

Sometimes the skin around a mole loses its color so the mole appears to be surrounded by a white ring. This is called a "halo nevus" and is harmless. We leave it alone. With time, the white ring often disappears.

Malignant melanoma, a rare cancerous growth that may resemble a mole, is dangerous and should be removed surgically. It seldom appears before the age of 20 years.

Treatment

Most moles are harmless and safe to ignore. Moles may be treated under the following conditions:

1. A mole that has bled, has an unusual shape, is growing rapidly, or changing color noticeably is giving warning signs of *possible* malignancy.
2. A mole that is irritated by your clothing, comb, or razor is only a nuisance, but your doctor can remove it to prevent ongoing irritation.
3. A mole that is unsightly can be removed for "cosmetic reasons."

Treating a protruding mole is a simple procedure. After numbing the skin, the doctor removes the projecting part of the mole with scissors or a scalpel. He may, as a matter of course, send the removed portion to a laboratory for microscopic examination. The wound heals to leave a flat mole, but the color generally remains the same. As a rule, dark moles leave dark spots.

Complete destruction of a mole requires removing the full thickness of skin. The resulting scar may be more noticeable than the mole was. For that reason, I avoid complete removal of facial moles and urge you to forget about treatment. Instead, think of moles as beauty spots.

Moles sometimes grow annoyingly coarse hair, and it may be safely removed by shaving or plucking. Permanent removal of the hair, which has roots deep within the skin, requires electrolysis or complete surgical excision of the mole.

Summary

The great majority of moles are harmless and best ignored. Protuberant moles that annoy you can easily be converted into flat moles by simple office surgery. Bleeding, rapid growth, unusual appearance, or sudden change in a mole are urgent reasons to consult your physician.

Molluscum contagiosum

What is molluscum contagiosum?

Molluscum contagiosum consists of small, harmless skin growths caused by a virus. They resemble pimples at first. Later, when they enlarge, they often have a waxy, pinkish look and a small central pit.

Molluscum contagiosum can be spread from person to person by direct skin contact. It is harmless and never turns cancerous.

Treatment

There is no single perfect treatment of molluscum contagiosum since we are unable to kill the virus. Individual lesions can be destroyed by a blistering agent, by liquid nitrogen, or by superficial surgical removal.

Sometimes new lesions will form while existing ones are being destroyed. New growths should be treated when they become large enough to be seen.

Molluscum lesions may become red and sore when the body tries to reject the virus. Sometimes a rash appears around the growths. These symptoms are harmless and can be safely ignored.

Nickel allergy

What causes nickel allergy?

Nickel allergy, like other allergies, may develop at any age. We don't know why some persons become allergic to nickel while others never do. Once you've become allergic to nickel, you're likely to have the allergy for many years.

Nickel allergy is especially common in women. It often prevents them from wearing jewelry. Persons allergic to nickel may break out from contact with nickel-containing or nickel-plated objects such as bracelets, earrings, zippers, bra hooks, and metal eyeglass frames. Although many coins contain nickel, they don't usually cause rashes.

Some persons are highly allergic to nickel and get a rash from even brief contact with nickel-containing metals, while others break out only after a long period of skin contact with nickel. All jewelry contains nickel; there's less nickel in 14- or 18-karat gold jewelry than in inexpensive costume jewelry. As a result, many are able to wear high-quality gold jewelry but break out when they wear cheaper costume jewelry.

Persons allergic to nickel can touch stainless steel without trouble—unless it's nickel-plated. Therefore, you don't have to worry about contact with stainless-steel instruments, tools, sinks, cutlery, or cooking utensils.

Treatment

Nickel-allergy rashes usually clear up once contact with nickel-containing metal is stopped and a cortisone medicine is applied to the rash. *Preventing* nickel-contact rashes means avoiding skin contact with nickel-containing metals. This may be awkward, especially as far as wearing jewelry is concerned. When you want to wear your wedding ring or other "essential" jewelry, please try this compromise approach: Wear the jewelry only for short periods of time when you're away from home, and apply a cortisone cream to your skin before putting your jewelry on.

If your ears are pierced, you can obtain hypoallergenic earrings from companies such as H&A Enterprises, Inc., 143-19 25th Avenue, Whitestone, N.Y. 11357. Write and ask for a catalog.

Desensitization

There's no way to desensitize a person with nickel allergy with shots, pills, or any other method. Nickel allergy stays on for years, although sometimes it gradually becomes less severe.

Pityriasis rosea

What causes pityriasis rosea?
Pityriasis rosea is a common, harmless skin disease. The cause is unknown, but we do know that:

1. Pityriasis rosea is *not* contagious.
2. Pityriasis rosea clears up in about three to six weeks, sometimes a little longer. When clear, the skin returns to its normal appearance. There will be no scars.
3. Pityriasis rosea is not related to foods, medicines, or nervous upsets.
4. Pityriasis rosea always disappears by itself.
5. A single scaling spot often appears 1 to 20 days before the general rash. The rash covers mainly the trunk but may spread to the thighs, upper arms, and neck. Pityriasis rosea usually avoids the face, although sometimes a few spots spread to the cheeks.
6. Second attacks of pityriasis rosea are rare.

Treatment
Nature always cures this disorder—sometimes slowly. Treatment doesn't speed the cure. The rash of pityriasis rosea is irritated by soap; bathe or shower with plain water. This rash makes the skin dry; it helps to put a thin coating of bath oil on your freshly dried skin after a shower or bath.

   If the rash itches, treatment with a cortisone usually brings prompt relief. The cortisone does not cure pityriasis rosea; it will only make you more comfortable while getting over the rash.

Poison ivy/poison oak allergy (*Rhus* allergy)

What causes poison ivy rash?

Poison ivy and poison oak rashes are caused by allergy to the juices of these plants—called *Rhus* plants. You don't have to come in direct contact with the leaves, roots, or branches of *Rhus* plants to get the rash. The plant juice can reach your skin indirectly when you touch clothing or a pet that carries the plant juice.

Like other allergies, *Rhus* allergy is acquired; you're not born with it. While some lucky people never become allergic to *Rhus* plants, most persons become sensitized at some time and remain allergic. Unfortunately, there's no way to desensitize persons allergic to *Rhus* plants. The many drops, tablets, and injections that supposedly produce immunity are of little value. Some have caused unpleasant side effects. I don't recommend them.

Contagion

Your poison ivy rash is not contagious. The fluid in the blisters does not spread the rash. *Rhus* rash doesn't appear immediately after exposure to the plant juice, but only after a time called the latent period. This latent period between exposure to the plant and appearance of the rash may be as short as four hours or as long as 10 days, depending on individual sensitivity and the amount of plant contact. Sometimes more rash appears after treatment has begun. These new patches are areas that had a longer latent period.

Treatment

Rhus rashes are self-limited—sooner or later they clear up without treatment. Letting nature take its course is reasonable with mild *Rhus* rash, but severe rashes need treatment to ease the misery and disability they cause. Cortisones taken by mouth are dramatically effective in treating *Rhus* rash. It's safe to take these drugs for a short period (two or three weeks). If you have a peptic ulcer, high blood pressure, or diabetes, you should take cortisone only under close medical supervision.

Medicines taken by mouth are needed during the early, severe stages of *Rhus* rash, since remedies applied to your skin don't penetrate deeply enough. Compress crusted or oozing areas for 15 minutes twice daily with a mixture of two to four tablespoons of white vinegar in two quarts of cool water. Ice packs or cold showers or baths will temporarily relieve your itching. Some persons find they get more relief by putting very hot water on the itchy areas. After 12 to 24 hours, cortisone will control your rash and itch.

Improvement in your rash should be prompt and steady. It depends on getting enough cortisone. If you don't improve steadily, please telephone this office so I can modify your treatment. Treatment changes can usually be managed by telephone; you probably won't have to make a return visit.

When the swelling has gone down, cortisone cream or ointment will help your rash heal. You will be given a prescription for a cortisone cream. Please don't use it until the swelling is down and blistering has stopped, as otherwise you'll waste it. Don't put anything on your rash except the prescription cream, water, and the vinegar-water mixture. You may bathe or shower as usual; keep the water as cool as you can stand and don't use soap on your rash, as it irritates.

Prevention

The only way to prevent *Rhus* rash is to avoid contact with the plant juice. It's traditional advice to wash with strong soap after poison ivy or poison oak exposure. This does no harm, but in order to prevent a rash, you have to wash within 15 minutes of exposure. If you can do so, simple washing with water and mild soap will effectively remove any plant juice from clothing, pets, or tools. Strong soaps are unnecessary. *Rhus* plants may cause rashes throughout the year. Roots and stems can cause a rash just as much as the leaves. If you can't recognize poison ivy or poison oak plants, have friends or neighbors point them out so you can avoid them.

Care after superficial skin surgery

The scab (crust) that covers your skin surgery is nature's bandage, and healing takes place beneath the scab. The scab will fall off by itself when healing is nearly complete. Please follow these directions:

1. Paint the scab twice daily with ordinary rubbing alcohol. Use a cotton-tipped applicator. Allow the alcohol to evaporate.
2. Leave the scab uncovered overnight.
3. During the day, either leave the scab uncovered or cover it with a Band-Aid, whichever you prefer.
4. You may apply makeup or powder over the scab.
5. It's best to keep the scab dry. You may get it wet temporarily, provided you dry the scab gently afterward. When swimming, protect the scab with a Band-Aid. Be sure to remove the wet Band-Aid when you come out of the water.

6. If the scab cracks or oozes, buy a tube of _____ ointment (no prescription needed) and apply it thinly five times a day.
7. If the skin around the wound becomes red, swollen, and painful, you may have an infected wound. Call me promptly.

Wound care

Following these directions will speed up the healing process.

1. While the wound is raw or oozing, cover it with a Band-Aid to which you have applied a little Polysporin or bacitracin ointment (no prescription needed).
2. Polysporin and bacitracin ointments are two antibiotic ointments available without prescription. Antibiotic ointments prevent wound infection and keep the bandage from sticking to the wound surface.
3. When washing your skin, avoid the wound area. There's no harm in getting the bandage temporarily wet; if you do, apply a fresh bandage along with a little antibiotic ointment.
4. Wipe off any pus on the wound surface with a clean paper tissue (Kleenex) when you change your bandage.
5. Wounds may bleed. Bleeding will usually stop if you apply pressure over the bandage for 10 minutes by the clock.
6. When the wound has healed or is covered by a dry crust, remove the bandage and leave the wound exposed. Any sticky tape remnants around the wound can be removed with a cotton-tipped applicator moistened with nail-polish remover.
7. If the skin around the wound becomes red, swollen, and painful, you may have an infected wound. Call me promptly.

Care of the sutured (stitched) wound

Keep your wound dry and covered with a bandage for the first two days. If you change the bandage, use sterile gauze or a Band-Aid to which you've applied a small amount of Polysporin or bacitracin (antibiotic) ointment. No prescription is needed. After two days you may get the bandage wet. Remove a wet bandage promptly and replace it with a dry bandage spread with antibiotic ointment.

Removal of the stitches is painless and is done 2 to 10 days after surgery. The wound will then be left open, or I may use tape to protect it and keep it closed. You can get the tape wet. Leave it on until it becomes loose—in 4 to 10 days.

Discomfort and swelling are usual between 6 and 20 hours after surgery. If they're annoying, take acetaminophen (Tylenol) or a similar *non*-aspirin mild painkiller. Avoid aspirin and medicines containing aspirin for two days after surgery, since they may cause easy bleeding. If the pain continues or if severe discomfort or swelling develops, please call this office promptly.

Bleeding sometimes occurs after surgery. You can ignore a little bleeding, but you should control heavier bleeding by putting firm pressure on the wound with Kleenex or a clean cloth. Do this, without stopping, for 10 minutes by the clock. Should the amount of bleeding concern you, or if it's not controlled after continuous pressure for 10 minutes, please call this office.

Care of wounds closed with dissolving stitches

Your wound has been closed with stitches that dissolve by themselves. They will fall out as the wound heals. They do not need to be removed by a physician.

The wound is covered with two different dressings. Next to the skin is a tape support that *must be left in place*. On top of the tape support is a gauze bandage.

1. Keep the wound dry for two days. Thereafter, you may get it wet.
2. Remove the gauze bandage tomorrow. Underneath the gauze dressing is a tape support. *Do not remove the tape support.*
3. Leave the tape support, which helps the wound to heal, in place until

_____ or longer, if possible. After that, if the tape loosens, you may gently remove it.
4. When the tape is off, remove any remaining tape adhesive with nail-polish remover or acetone.
5. From 6 to 20 hours after surgery, you may expect some discomfort and swelling. You may take a mild painkiller such as acetaminophen (Tylenol). If the pain continues or if severe discomfort or swelling develops, please call this office promptly.
6. Bleeding sometimes occurs after surgery. You can ignore a little bleeding, but you should control heavy bleeding by putting firm pressure on the wound with a clean paper tissue or cloth *for 10 minutes by the clock.* If the amount of bleeding concerns you, or if it's not controlled after continuous pressure for 10 minutes, please call this office.

Liquid nitrogen treatment

Liquid nitrogen is a cold, liquified gas with a temperature of 196° below zero Celsius ($-321°$ Fahrenheit). It's used to freeze and destroy superficial skin growths such as warts and keratoses. Liquid nitrogen causes stinging and mild pain while the growth is being frozen and then thaws. The discomfort lasts less than five minutes.

Some hours after liquid nitrogen treatment your skin will become swollen and red; later on it may blister. Then a scab (crust) will form. It will fall off by itself in one to three weeks. The skin growth will come off along with the scab, leaving healthy new skin.

If your growth required deep freezing to remove, there may be considerable blistering and swelling, especially if your hands or eyelids were treated. The blisters and swelling are part of the treatment and will gradually heal by themselves.

No special care is needed after liquid nitrogen treatment. Just ignore it. You can wash your skin as usual and use makeup or other cosmetics. If clothing irritates the area, cover it with a small bandage (Band-Aid).

Sometimes liquid nitrogen treatment fails. If the growth is not cured by liquid nitrogen, please make a return appointment.

Pruritus ani (rectal itch)

What causes pruritus ani?
Itching of the skin about the anus (opening of the rectum) is a common complaint. The skin is exposed to irritating digestive products in the stool; this may lead to an itchy rash, especially when stools are frequent. Often the rash is worsened by vigorous use of toilet tissue or scrubbing with soap and water.

Anal itching is usually an isolated skin complaint in otherwise healthy persons, but in some it's part of a disorder involving other areas of the skin. Whether pruritus ani is an isolated problem or part of another skin disorder, irritation from stools and from cleansing after bowel movements keeps the rash going. You may find that coffee and spicy foods make it worse. These foods irritate the digestive tract and increase the number of stools or amount of mucus (liquid) secreted from the rectum.

Treatment
Treatment is intended to reduce irritation of the anal skin. Unfortunately, it's impossible to eliminate all irritation, since it's impossible to avoid contact of the stool with inflamed skin. Careful, thorough, gentle cleansing after bowel movements is *very* important. Moisten toilet paper with lukewarm water, as dry toilet paper doesn't cleanse as well as wet and also irritates your skin. Never use soap on the anal area. Cleansing with plain water, in either the shower or bathtub, will do the job.

You will be given a soothing preparation, which you should apply thinly with your fingertips after each bowel movement, at bedtime, and at other times during the day as directed. *Do not apply any other remedy, suppository, or medicine to your rash.* Only the prescription medicine, water, moist toilet paper, and clean underwear should ever touch inflamed anal skin.

Pruritus ani is frequently stubborn and requires months of local medication and gentle skin care. Pruritus ani often comes back. Therefore, don't throw your medicines away when you are free from itching, but keep them on hand in case your trouble returns. Some persons need to continue using the medication once or twice daily indefinitely, since the itching returns whenever they stop. Anyone who has had pruritus ani should, for at least one year, keep soap off the anal skin and use only wet toilet paper for cleansing after bowel movements. If the medicine no longer controls your rash, please return.

Psoriasis

What causes psoriasis?

Psoriasis is a common skin disorder affecting about 1 in 40 persons. In the United States more than 4 million people have psoriasis. The cause of psoriasis is not known. Many persons with psoriasis have blood relatives with this disorder, so heredity plays a role.

In psoriasis, areas of the skin grow much faster than normal and form red, scaling patches. The scalp, elbows, and knees are the most common sites, but almost any part of the skin may become involved. Fortunately, psoriasis is only a skin condition and does not affect your general health. (In rare cases it may be associated with arthritis.) Psoriasis is a problem because it itches and is unsightly. Psoriasis is *not* contagious.

Psoriasis usually begins in young adulthood, although it can start in childhood or first appear in old age. In most cases psoriasis is mild and is limited to a few areas of the body. In a small percentage of cases, large areas of the body may become involved. Psoriasis is unpredictable: Patches may clear up by themselves and even disappear for months or years.

Treatment

You will be given detailed, individualized instructions for treatment of your psoriasis. Treatment is temporarily effective, and may need to be continued for quite a while. You will find it reassuring to know that (1) diet does *not* affect psoriasis, (2) psoriasis will *not* cause your hair to fall out, and (3) psoriasis is *not* caused by nerves. A nervous upset sometimes worsens psoriasis—just as nervous upsets may worsen any illness.

If you have psoriasis of the scalp, it helps to wash your hair often. A medicated shampoo isn't necessary. Some other treatments used in psoriasis are these:

1. Moderate sunlight exposure is often helpful. Don't get sunburned, since psoriasis may settle in areas of injured skin.
2. Ultraviolet light by itself often helps psoriasis. Ultraviolet light is even more effective when used with tar or anthralin.
3. Cytotoxic drugs such as methotrexate, given by mouth or injection, are used only for very severe psoriasis. *Cytotoxic* means *poisonous to cells,* and these drugs are used only with special precautions.
4. PUVA treatment combines a psoralen (an internal medicine) with ultraviolet light A (PUVA = *P*soralen + *U*ltra*V*iolet *A*). This therapy is available only at certain centers, as it requires specialized light equipment. While PUVA is an effective treatment for extensive psoriasis, like all other treatments it is only of temporary benefit.

While psoriasis is an unsightly nuisance, it should not prevent you from leading a full, active life.

Rosacea

What is rosacea?
Rosacea is a fairly common annoying face rash of adults. The rash of rosacea has red areas and pimples. It's especially noticeable on the nose, mid-forehead, and chin. Rosacea pimples resemble the acne pimples of teen-agers, and years ago rosacea used to be called acne rosacea. Rosacea is only a skin condition and is not related to your general health. Sometimes eye irritation occurs in rosacea. While in some persons rosacea causes mild itching or burning, its unsightly appearance is the usual reason for treating it.

What causes it?
The cause of rosacea is unknown. Rosacea is stubborn and often lasts for years. Foods or beverages that cause facial flushing, such as alcohol, spicy foods, and hot soups and drinks, may make rosacea *temporarily* more noticeable.

Treatment
Antibiotics taken by mouth are usually effective in controlling rosacea. Why antibiotics work is not known, since rosacea is *not an infectious disease.* Treatment only controls rosacea. Most persons with this condition need to continue taking antibiotics for months to years.

Scabies

What causes scabies?

Scabies—also known as "the itch"—is an intensely itching rash caused by a tiny mite (bug) that lives in the skin. Since it is only $\frac{1}{60}$ inch long, the scabies mite is almost impossible to see without magnification.

The rash usually involves the hands, wrists, breasts, genital area, and waistline. In severe cases scabies can spread to almost the entire body—never to the face. Scabies often resembles other rashes. The only way to find out whether you have scabies is for a doctor to scrape off a piece of skin and examine it under a microscope.

Contagion

Scabies is contagious—it's transmitted by close personal contact. All members of your family, and any sexual partners you may have, should be treated *at the same time*. Scabies is *not* spread by clothes or bedding; there's no need to sterilize sheets, towels, blankets, or clothing.

Treatment

Treatment consists of applying a mite-killing medication to your skin. Follow directions exactly. Apply the medicine to your *entire* skin from the neck down, not just to the itching areas. Rub the medicine thoroughly into your hands and wrists. *Do not wash your hands for eight hours. Do not apply the medicine longer than directed,* as it will irritate your skin.

Your itching and rash may continue even though all the mites have been killed. This results from allergy to the mites and is called postscabetic dermatitis. Postscabetic dermatitis is *not* scabies, and requires special treatment. Don't try to treat it with the mite-killing medicine.

The itching rash of scabies usually clears up in two to six weeks if (1) you carry out your treatment exactly as instructed and (2) all close personal and sexual contacts are treated at the same time.

Seborrheic keratoses

What causes seborrheic keratoses?

Seborrheic keratoses are harmless, common skin growths that first appear during adult life. As time goes by, more growths appear. Some persons have a very large number of them. Seborrheic keratoses appear on both covered and uncovered parts of the body; they are not caused by sunlight. The tendency to develop seborrheic keratoses is inherited.

Seborrheic keratoses are harmless and never become malignant. They begin as slightly raised, light brown spots. Gradually they thicken and take on a rough, warty surface. They slowly darken and may turn black. These color changes are harmless. Seborrheic keratoses are superficial and look as if they were stuck on the skin. Persons who have had several seborrheic keratoses can usually recognize this type of benign growth. However, if you are concerned or unsure about any growth, consult me.

Treatment

Seborrheic keratoses can easily be removed in the office. The only reason for removing a seborrheic keratosis is your wish to get rid of it—if it's unsightly, itches, or annoys you by rubbing against your clothes.

Sunlight and your skin

Why avoid the sun?
Sunlight permanently damages skin. Ordinary sun exposure during tanning and outdoor sports causes permanent skin changes. These changes build up over the years, so that even moderate repeated sun exposure causes visible skin damage. Most of the wrinkling, roughening, and freckling that appears on the face, hands, and arms of white adults comes from sun damage, not age. You can see this if you compare less sun-exposed areas, such as your abdomen or the undersides of your arms, with sun-exposed areas such as your face, neck, or upper surfaces of your arms. The natural coloration of your skin—pigment—protects you from the damaging effects of sunlight. Persons with fair skin—who have little pigmentation—are more prone to sun damage than dark-skinned individuals.

The skin-damaging effects of sunlight
The skin-damaging effects of sunlight gradually lead to roughening, freckling, and wrinkling. Many people in their 30s and 40s are unhappy because their wrinkled, roughened, sun-damaged skin makes them appear 10 or 15 years older. Unfortunately, there's no way to undo these changes. Young people should realize that they'll ultimately pay a very steep price for the temporary glamour of a deep suntan.

A more serious effect of sun damage is skin cancer. Sun damage is the chief cause of skin cancer. Here again, fair-skinned individuals are much more susceptible. Skin cancer rarely occurs in blacks. As you might expect, skin cancer tends to occur on sun-exposed areas such as the face, neck, shoulders, and arms. While skin cancers can usually be removed by minor surgery in a doctor's office, it's better to prevent them.

Ultraviolet rays—the invisible enemy
Sunlight contains both ordinary, harmless, visible light and shorter, invisible light rays called ultraviolet light. Tanning, burning, and skin damage from sunlight are caused by ultraviolet rays. Since ultraviolet rays produce both tanning and skin damage, it's impossible to tan "safely" and avoid permanent skin damage. Discussions on sunbathing that describe "safe" tanning refer to the avoidance of sunburn. By proper timing, most persons can get a deep tan without a sunburn. However, no one can get a tan without some skin damage.

Sun-protective measures

There are two basic ways of protecting your skin from the damaging effects of ultraviolet rays: (1) by blocking out all light with an opaque material such as clothing and (2) by using a chemical sunscreen that selectively absorbs ultraviolet rays. Blocking out all light with clothing is most effective. Certain sun protectives depend on the same principle. They coat the skin with a paintlike pigment that mechanically blocks light. They work well, but they're messy and rather unsightly.

There are also many clear sunscreens that absorb ultraviolet light. These "clean" sunscreens contain either PABA (para-aminobenzoic acid) or a benzophenone compound. Some of the PABA-containing sunscreens are taken up by the skin and will provide some protection in the water—provided they're applied *one or two hours before swimming.* An occasional person is allergic to PABA or its derivatives, so please try PABA-type sunscreens on a small area of skin before spreading it all over your body. The other chemical class of sun protectives, the benzophenones, rarely cause skin allergy. Benzophenones wash off, however, and therefore do not protect swimmers. Some benzophenones have a bitter taste that can be annoying when applied near the mouth.

There are many sun protectives on the market. The better ones are labeled with a number called the sun-protective factor (SPF). The higher the SPF number, the better the protection. The best sunscreens have an SPF of 15, and are what you should use.

Water removes most sunscreens. Remember to put on another coat of sunscreen after swimming or bathing. If you're sweating heavily, use some more sunscreen every hour or two. If you're in very bright sunlight, it's wise to protect your skin as much as possible with clothing (long sleeves, gloves, wide-brimmed hats) and use one of the "clean" chemical sunscreens on the parts of your skin exposed to the sun.

Protect your lips from sun damage. The darker lipstick shades are effective for women. Men—and women who don't wear lipstick—should use an ultraviolet-absorbing lip pomade. Women can use makeup with a sun protective. The sun protective should be applied first, then the makeup. The makeup itself—especially if heavily colored—provides some sun protection.

You should aim to minimize sun exposure, not avoid it. Being outdoors is fun and healthful; *don't* let fear of sun damage keep you inside during sunny weather. *Do* use sun protectives when enjoying sports or a walk in the sun.

Tetracycline treatment of acneiform eruptions

Tetracycline, an antibiotic taken internally, controls acne in two out of three patients. Tetracycline usually controls rosacea and perioral dermatitis. Since tetracycline does not cure but only suppresses these skin disorders, the antibiotic has to be continued until the disease runs its course. It may be necessary to continue taking tetracycline for months or years. Long-term treatment with tetracycline is remarkably safe; we have had over 30 years' experience with tetracycline.

Dosage

Patients differ in the amount of tetracycline they need. You'll start with a full daily dose of tetracycline to see if it controls your skin problem. When a full dose of tetracycline has controlled your skin problem, you'll gradually reduce the amount of tetracycline to find the smallest number of pills that will keep it under control. This minimum amount needed to control your skin problem may be as little as one pill every other day or as much as four or more pills a day.

In determining the smallest number of pills needed to control your skin disorder, you will gradually reduce your dose by one pill a day. It's best to stay at each dosage level for four to six weeks, since there's a lag period of one to three weeks between the change in dosage and its effect on your skin. You should gradually reduce the amount of tetracycline until your eruption becomes worse; then return to the previous higher dosage and continue on it to control the pimples or rash. You have now determined the minimum dose you require. After a few months, try again to lower the amount of tetracycline by one pill a day.

It's all right to change your daily dose of tetracycline if you do it systematically and gradually. For example, many teen-agers find that during summer they need less tetracycline than in winter because summer sunshine helps their acne. They gradually decrease their tetracycline in spring and summer as their acne improves, and then increase it again in fall and winter as their acne worsens. Young women may find that they can control premenstrual acne flare-ups by increasing their tetracycline doses for 7 to 10 days before the expected flare-ups. Changes in dosage should be systematic; do *not* change the dose from day to day.

Side effects

Even when taken for months or years, tetracycline has few side effects. Tetracycline makes persons more sensitive to sunlight; this effect depends on the amount taken. On one or two tablets a day, few people have problems even in sunny summer weather. On four or more a day, many persons sunburn very easily. If you find that you sunburn more easily while taking tetracycline, protect yourself with sunscreens or sun blockers, or wear protective clothing. Not only the face but the hands, fingernails, and other exposed skin areas need protection from sunlight. In women, tetracycline occasionally produces an annoying genital itch because of its effect on the bacteria of the vagina. If this harmless but annoying side effect occurs, please call my office.

   CAUTION: *Tetracycline should not be taken during pregnancy.*

Dosage reduction schedule

Please use the following schedule to determine the smallest dose of tetracycline you need to control your skin problem.

1. On _____ reduce your tetracycline pills to _____ pills on arising and _____ in the evening.
2. If your eruption is well controlled on _____ pills a day, on _____ reduce to _____ on arising and _____ in the evening.
3. If _____ pills a day keeps your eruption under good control, on _____ decrease your daily dose by one pill.
4. When you're down to one pill a day, try reducing your dosage to one pill every other day. Then, if one pill every other day is enough, try stopping tetracycline, as you may not need it anymore.

   It's important to keep on reducing your dosage gradually until you start to break out—then continue taking the smallest dose that previously controlled your eruption.

Tinea cruris ("jock itch")

What causes tinea cruris?

"Jock itch" refers to any itching groin rash of men and is not a medical term. There are many causes for "jock itch"; when caused by a fungus, the rash is known as tinea cruris. The fungus causing tinea cruris is a microscopic plant that grows in the outer skin and prefers moisture. When this fungus infects the feet, it's called athlete's foot (tinea pedis).

Contagion

Fortunately, tinea cruris is not contagious. Direct person-to-person spreading is not a problem. The patient's own case of athlete's foot is the usual source of infection and reinfection of the groin.

Treatment

Tinea cruris is treated by applying the antifungal medicine _____ thinly three times a day with your fingertips. Spread the medicine on sparingly and massage it in gently until it disappears. To prevent recurrences, continue the antifungal medicine for two weeks after the rash has cleared up.

Apply nothing else to your groin except water. Cleanse your groin with plain water, since soap aggravates groin rashes.

Tinea cruris usually clears up promptly with antifungal medicines applied to the skin. If it doesn't, you may need two to three weeks of treatment with the antifungal antibiotic griseofulvin, taken by mouth.

Tinea cruris is only *one* cause of groin itching. If your rash does not improve, please return for further evaluation.

Prevention

Tinea cruris often comes back. Warmth and moisture encourage the fungus to grow. You can help prevent recurrences by drying thoroughly after bathing, wearing loose cotton underwear, and dusting a bland powder on your groin once or twice daily. After swimming, put on dry clothes right away; don't stay long in a wet swimsuit.

Tinea versicolor

What causes tinea versicolor?

Tinea versicolor is a harmless skin disorder caused by a germ living on normal skin. Usually this germ—which all of us have on our skin—grows sparsely and is not visible. In some individuals it grows more actively. This causes the slightly scaling patches on the trunk, neck, or arms known as tinea versicolor. On untanned skin tinea versicolor rash is a pink to coppery tan. On tanned skin the tinea versicolor patches are lighter, since tanning doesn't occur in the rash areas. The failure to tan is temporary; the skin tans normally after the rash has cleared up.

Tinea versicolor is *not* contagious. Tinea versicolor is more common in hot, humid climates and often comes back in the summertime.

Treatment

Treatment with one overnight application of selenium sulfide suspension is usually effective. At bedtime, massage the medicine thoroughly into the affected area. Spread the medicine over large areas: If you have spots on your chest, apply medicine to your entire trunk. The next morning, scrub off all the medicine in the shower. Usually a single treatment will make tinea versicolor gradually disappear over the next few weeks. If you still have the rash one month after the treatment, repeat it *once.* If the rash hasn't gone away by one month after the second overnight treatment with selenium sulfide, please return.

There are other ways of treating tinea versicolor. Double-strength Whitfield's ointment (available without prescription) applied very thinly at bedtime for 10 to 14 days is often effective. A simpler, cleaner medication is 50 percent propylene glycol in water applied nightly for several weeks. Prescription antifungal ointments such as miconazole (Monistat) or clotrimazole (Lotrimin, Mycelex) clear up tinea versicolor but are expensive.

Unfortunately, tinea versicolor—being caused by a normal skin inhabitant—tends to recur. When it does, repeat the previously successful treatment. If recurrences are frequent, you may be able to prevent them by treating your skin once every three months with selenium sulfide overnight.

Warts

What causes warts?

Warts are harmless skin growths caused by a virus. Warts can grow on any part of the body. Their appearance depends on their location. On the face and tops of the hands warts protrude, while on such pressure areas as the palms of the hands and soles of the feet they're pushed inward. Warts on the bottoms of the feet (called plantar warts) grow inward from the pressure of standing and walking and are often painful. Warts have a rough surface on which tiny dark specks can often be seen.

Warts are common and can be a nuisance. They may bleed if injured. Warts never turn cancerous.

Since warts are caused by a virus, they are slightly contagious. Warts may spread on the body since a wart is the source of a virus that can seed other areas. We don't know why some persons get warts easily while others never get them. There's no way to prevent warts.

People have been trying to cure warts for thousands of years. The "success" of folk remedies for warts is due to the fact that warts often disappear by themselves, especially in young children. This spontaneous disappearance is less common in older children and adults.

Treatment

There is no single perfect treatment of warts, since we are unable to kill the virus. Treatment consists of destroying the wart. Warts can be destroyed with surgery, by freezing with liquid nitrogen, or with chemicals. The treatment to be used on your warts depends on their location and size, your type of skin, and my professional medical judgment.

Sometimes new warts will form while existing ones are being destroyed. All we can do is treat the new warts when they become large enough to be seen.

No matter what treatment is used, warts occasionally fail to disappear. Warts may return weeks or months after an apparent cure. Don't become concerned if a wart recurs. Please make an appointment for a return visit. The treatment will be repeated, or a different method will be used to destroy the wart.

Plantar warts

What causes plantar warts?

Plantar warts are ordinary warts of the sole, or plantar surface, of the foot. Since plantar warts are on a pressure area, they grow inward and are often tender and painful. Like other warts, plantar warts are caused by a virus and are harmless.

Treatment

There are many ways of treating plantar warts. All involve destroying the warts. So far we don't have a perfect treatment for plantar warts. I prefer to treat plantar warts by destroying them chemically. This treatment is painless and will let you engage in your usual activities. It usually succeeds if carried out according to instructions. It will take several weeks or months.

You will be given a prescription that is to be used as follows:

1. At bedtime, put a tiny amount of wart-destroying medicine exactly on your warts with _____
Put the medicine only on the warts, as it may irritate normal skin.
2. After applying the medicine, cover your warts with adhesive tape. Use the old-fashioned fabric type of adhesive tape. The tape keeps your skin moist. The moisture softens the surface of the warts so the medicine will penetrate. It's all right to get the tape wet.
3. In the morning, take off the adhesive tape. If your skin tears when you remove the tape, loosen the tape by painting nail-polish remover (use a cotton-tipped applicator) between your skin and the tape.
4. After a few days the outside of the warts will start to turn gray. This means the chemical has begun to destroy them. Scrape this gray wart tissue off with the point of a metal nail file every second or third day. Do the scraping after a bath or shower has softened the warts' surface. Be sure to remove *every bit* of dead wart tissue; otherwise it will keep the wart-destroying medicine from reaching the living tissue underneath. Sometimes a small curved scissors or a pumice stone helps in removing the dead wart tissue. Whatever you use for scraping your warts should not be used for anything else, because warts are somewhat contagious.
5. If the warts become sore, stop the treatment for a few days.
6. If you don't see much progress after two to three weeks, try leaving the tape on until noon, or even longer. Stubborn warts may need to be covered continuously with tape.

7. If your plantar warts hurt when you stand or walk, wear a pad cut out of *Dr. Scholl's Adhesive Foam* (available without prescription). Cut a hole (or holes) corresponding to where the warts are. This will take the pressure off the warts.

8. Continue the treatment until you believe the warts are gone. If you can see the lines of your skin crossing the treated area, the warts are probably gone. If it turns out that after you stop treatment the warts are still there—it happens— start treating them again until you feel more certain that the warts have gone away.

9. If necessary, continue the treatment for four months. If the warts haven't been destroyed after four months of treatment, return; a different approach will be used.

10. In case the warts become painful or infected, return at once.

Chemical destruction of warts

Chemical destruction of warts is a painless alternative to office surgery. Chemical destruction is also used when there are many warts and surgical removal is not practical.

You will put a medicine on your wart at bedtime, then cover it with tape. The tape covering holds the medicine in place and helps it penetrate into the wart. The medicine gradually eats the wart away. Dead wart tissue builds up on the surface; you *must* scrape it off. Continue the treatment until all traces of the wart have been destroyed. This usually takes one to three months.

Here are the steps:

1. At bedtime, put a tiny amount of wart-destroying medicine exactly on your wart with

---

Put the medicine *only on the wart,* as it will irritate normal skin.

2. After applying the medicine, cover the wart with waterproof adhesive tape. The tape keeps your skin moist. The moisture softens the surface of the wart so the medicine will penetrate more deeply. It's all right to get the tape wet.

3. In the morning, take off the adhesive tape. If your skin tears when you remove the tape, loosen the tape by painting nail-polish remover (use a cotton-tipped applicator) between your skin and the tape.

4. After a few days the outside of the wart will start to turn gray. That means the chemical has begun to destroy the wart. Scrape this gray wart tissue off with the point of a metal nail file every second or third day. Do the scraping after a bath or shower has softened the wart's surface. Be sure to remove *every bit* of dead wart tissue; otherwise it will keep the wart-destroying medicine from reaching the living tissue underneath. Sometimes a small curved scissors or a pumice stone helps in removing the dead tissue. Whatever you use for scraping your wart should not be used for anything else, as warts are somewhat contagious.

5. If the wart becomes sore, stop the treatment for a few days.

6. If you don't see much progress after two to three weeks, try leaving the tape on until noon, or even longer. Stubborn warts may need to be covered continuously with tape.

7. Continue the treatment until you believe the wart is gone. If it turns out that the wart is still there after you stop treatment, start treating it again until you feel more certain it has gone away.

8. If after three months the wart hasn't been destroyed, please return for a re-evaluation.